Reviving Iran,

A Journey Towards Health and Hope

Written by

Ali R. Rahimi, M.D., FACP, AGSF

ENDURING POWER OF HOPE AND JUSTICE

Increasing Awareness and Global Perspectives

Contents

Dedication

I dedicate this book to the resilient and courageous Iranian people, this book is a heartfelt tribute to the freedom fighters, poets, artists, singers, students, and protesters who have faced unimaginable hardships. It is a solemn acknowledgment of those who have been unjustly jailed, and those who have tragically lost their eyes and their lives in the pursuit of justice and freedom. Above all, it is a tribute to their brave mothers, who have stood as pillars of strength and resilience, inspiring hope amidst darkness. May this book serve as a testament to their unwavering spirit and as a beacon of solidarity with the Iranian people in pursuing democracy.

Hope

Hope, an ethereal force that permeates our lives, is a beacon of light amid the darkest of times. It is an intangible yet potent emotion that fuels our dreams, ignites our passions, and propels us forward despite adversity. In this essay, we will explore the profound significance of hope, its transformative influence on individuals and societies, and how it shapes our perception of the world.

1. The Essence of Hope:

Hope is an intrinsic part of being human, an emotion that arises from our innate desire for progress, growth, and happiness. It is the belief that positive change is possible, even in the face of daunting challenges. Hope encompasses optimism, resilience, and the unwavering faith that tomorrow can be better than today.

2. Nurturing the Human Spirit:

Hope has an extraordinary ability to uplift and inspire. It kindles a sense of possibility within us, infusing us with the courage to persevere through hardships. It empowers individuals to overcome obstacles, driving them to take action and strive for their goals. Hope nurtures the human spirit, invigorating us with renewed purpose and determination.

3. A Catalyst for Change:

Throughout history, hope has been at the forefront of transformative movements. It has fueled social, political, and cultural revolutions, mobilizing communities to challenge injustice and envision a better future. From the civil rights movement to the fight against oppression, hope has united people in the pursuit of a more equitable and compassionate world.

4. Hope as a Healing Force:

In times of personal crisis or collective trauma, hope becomes an indispensable source of solace and healing. It offers solace to those burdened by grief, reminding them that life can regain its vibrancy. Hope provides comfort to those battling illness, reminding them that recovery is possible. It is a balm for wounded souls, rejuvenating them with the promise of brighter days ahead.

5. Inspiring Creativity and Innovation:

Hope unleashes the boundless potential of the human mind. It fosters creativity, as it encourages individuals to envision new possibilities and explore uncharted territories. In times of uncertainty, hope fuels innovation, pushing us to find ingenious solutions to complex problems. It is the driving force behind groundbreaking inventions, artistic masterpieces, and scientific breakthroughs.

Hope, an intangible force that transcends boundaries and connects us all, is an indispensable facet of the human experience. It empowers individuals, transforms societies, and fuels progress. As we navigate the intricate tapestry of life, hope serves as a guiding light, reminding us that even in our darkest moments, there is always a glimmer of possibility. Let us embrace hope, nurture it within ourselves and others, and together, let it lead us toward a future brimming with promise and fulfillment.

Hope is an optimistic emotion that arises from a belief or desire for something better in the future. It is a feeling of expectation and anticipation, often accompanied by a sense of possibility and a willingness to act. Hope can fuel motivation, resilience, and determination to overcome obstacles and work towards goals. It is a fundamental human emotion that provides individuals with a sense of purpose, meaning, and the belief that positive change is possible.

While hope is generally associated with positive emotions, it can exist within a spectrum that encompasses both positive and negative outcomes. Hope can be seen as a positive emotion when it fuels optimism, resilience, and the belief in a better future. It provides motivation, inspiration, and a sense of purpose, leading individuals to work towards positive change.

However, hope can also possess a dual nature, as it can sometimes arise from negative circumstances or challenging situations. In such cases, hope may stem from a desire to overcome adversity or to find meaning in difficult experiences. This implies that hope can emerge from a place of pain, loss, or uncertainty.

Moreover, the outcome of hope is not always guaranteed to be positive. While hope can lead to positive outcomes, it can also result in disappointment, when expectations aren't met, or desired changes do not materialize. This aspect of hope, where it intersects with the risk of disappointment or failure, highlights the complexity of this emotion.

Ultimately, hope exists on a continuum, where it can be predominantly positive, but it can also encompass elements of uncertainty, vulnerability, and the potential for disappointment. It is the delicate balance between optimism and realism that shapes the nature and impact of hope in our lives.

Social and Political Plurality

Social and political plurality refers to the coexistence of diverse beliefs, opinions, and ideologies within a society or political system. It is an essential aspect of democratic societies, as it ensures that different voices are heard and considered in the decision-making process.

One of the key advantages of social and political plurality is that it encourages a healthy exchange of ideas and promotes critical thinking. When individuals from various backgrounds and perspectives engage in open dialogue, it leads to a richer understanding of complex issues and challenges. This diversity of thought can generate innovative solutions, as well as prevent the dominance of a single ideology or group.

Moreover, social and political plurality fosters inclusivity and equal representation. It recognizes that individuals have different needs, experiences, and aspirations, and aims to create a society where everyone's voice is valued and respected. This can lead to the recognition and protection of minority rights, and the promotion of social justice and equality.

Furthermore, social and political plurality plays a crucial role in holding power accountable. When multiple perspectives are present, it becomes more difficult for those in positions of authority to ignore dissenting opinions or act solely in their interests. Plurality ensures that decision-makers are exposed to a range of viewpoints, making it harder for them to abuse their power or make decisions that are not in the best interest of the broader society.

However, social and political plurality also presents challenges. It can lead to polarization and division, particularly when there is a lack of respectful and constructive dialogue. When individuals become entrenched in their own beliefs and refuse to consider alternative perspectives, it can hinder progress and hinder the search for common ground.

Furthermore, managing social and political plurality requires effective systems and institutions that can facilitate dialogue, mediate conflicts, and ensure fair representation for all. Without such mechanisms, plurality can lead to chaos and inequality, as certain groups may dominate the conversation or have their needs overlooked.

Social and political plurality refers to the coexistence of diverse beliefs, opinions, and ideologies within a society or political system. It is an essential aspect of democratic societies, as it ensures that different voices are heard and considered in the decision-making process.

One of the key advantages of social and political plurality is that it encourages a healthy exchange of ideas and promotes critical thinking. When individuals from various backgrounds and perspectives engage in open dialogue, it leads to a richer understanding of complex issues and challenges. This diversity of thought can generate innovative solutions, as well as prevent the dominance of a single ideology or group.

Moreover, social and political plurality fosters inclusivity and equal representation. It recognizes that individuals have different needs, experiences, and aspirations, and aims to create a society where everyone's voice is valued and respected. This can lead to the recognition and protection of minority rights, and the promotion of social justice and equality.

Furthermore, social and political plurality plays a crucial role in holding power accountable. When multiple perspectives are present, it becomes more difficult for those in positions of authority to ignore dissenting opinions or act solely in their own interests. Plurality ensures that decision-makers are exposed to a range of viewpoints, making it harder for them to abuse their power or make decisions that are not in the best interest of the broader society.

However, social and political plurality also presents challenges. It can lead to polarization and division, particularly when there is a lack of respectful and constructive dialogue. When individuals become entrenched in their own beliefs and refuse to consider alternative perspectives, it can hinder progress and hinder the search for common ground.

Furthermore, managing social and political plurality requires effective systems and institutions that can facilitate dialogue, mediate conflicts, and ensure fair representation for all. Without such mechanisms, plurality can lead to chaos and inequality, as certain groups may dominate the conversation or have their needs overlooked.

In conclusion, social and political plurality is vital for the functioning of democratic societies. It promotes diverse perspectives, critical thinking, and inclusivity. However, it also requires open-mindedness, respectful dialogue, and effective systems to navigate the challenges that arise. Striking a balance between embracing diversity and finding common ground is essential for a thriving and inclusive society. Social and political plurality is vital for the functioning of democratic societies. It promotes diverse perspectives, critical thinking, and inclusivity. However, it also requires open-mindedness, respectful dialogue, and effective systems to navigate the challenges that arise. Striking a balance between embracing diversity and finding common ground is essential for a thriving and inclusive society.

HOPE AND POLITICAL JUSTICE

Hope is an incredibly powerful emotion that can inspire individuals and communities to envision a better future. In the context of social and political plurality, hope plays a crucial role in fostering positive change and progress.

Social and political plurality refers to the coexistence of diverse perspectives, ideas, and beliefs within a society or political system. It recognizes that people have different backgrounds, experiences, and values, and encourages the inclusion and representation of these diverse voices.

Hope can be a driving force in promoting social and political plurality. It allows individuals to believe in the possibility of a more inclusive and equitable society, where different perspectives are respected and valued. Hope can motivate people to engage in dialogue, seek common ground, and work towards solutions that benefit a wide range of individuals.

Moreover, hope can help overcome challenges and obstacles that may arise in the pursuit of social and political plurality. It provides the resilience and determination needed to address systemic issues, navigate conflicts, and create meaningful change. When people have hope, they are more likely to persevere and find creative solutions to complex problems.

Hope also promotes empathy and understanding among individuals with differing viewpoints. By fostering an environment of hope, it becomes easier for people to engage in constructive conversations, listen to one another, and find shared values and goals. This paves the way for collaboration and cooperation, ultimately contributing to a more pluralistic and inclusive society.

To summarize, hope is a powerful catalyst for social and political plurality. It inspires individuals to imagine a better future, helps overcome challenges, and fosters empathy and understanding. By embracing hope, we can work towards creating a society that embraces diversity and respects the multitude of perspectives within it.

Yes, hope can indeed promote social and political plurality. Hope is a positive and motivating emotion that can inspire individuals and communities to come together and work towards a more inclusive and diverse society.

When people have hope, they believe in the possibility of change and progress. This belief can encourage individuals to engage in conversations and actions that promote social and political plurality. Hope can motivate people to seek common ground, listen to different perspectives, and find solutions that benefit a wider range of people.

Hope also plays a crucial role in overcoming challenges and obstacles that may arise in the pursuit of social and political plurality. It provides the resilience and determination needed to address systemic issues and navigate conflicts. When people have hope, they are more likely to persevere and find creative solutions to complex problems.

Furthermore, hope fosters empathy and understanding among individuals with differing viewpoints. It creates an environment where people are more willing to engage in constructive conversations, listen to one another, and find shared values and goals. This empathy and understanding are essential for building bridges of communication and cooperation, ultimately contributing to a more pluralistic and inclusive society.

Hope as a tool for political change and gain:

utilizing hope to promote social and political plurality involves taking proactive steps to inspire individuals and communities towards positive change. Here are some steps you can take:

1. Foster a sense of hope: Encourage discussions and initiatives that highlight positive examples of social and political progress. Share stories of individuals or groups who have made a difference, emphasizing the power of collective action and the potential for change.

2. Raise awareness and educate: Promote awareness about the importance of social and political plurality. Educate individuals about the benefits of diverse perspectives, inclusivity, and the value of respecting different opinions. Provide resources, workshops, or events that encourage learning and understanding.

3. Encourage open dialogue: Create spaces for open and respectful dialogue where individuals can express their viewpoints and engage in meaningful conversations. Foster an environment where people feel safe to share their opinions and listen to others without judgment. Encourage active listening and empathy.

4. Promote collaboration and cooperation: Encourage individuals from diverse backgrounds and with different perspectives to work together towards common goals. Facilitate partnerships and collaborations that bring together people with varied experiences and expertise. Highlight the power of collective action and the positive impact it can have.

5. Support grassroots initiatives: Identify and support grassroots movements, organizations, or community projects that promote social and political plurality. This can involve volunteering, donating, or actively participating in their activities. Amplify their voices and encourage others to get involved.

6. Engage in advocacy and policy change: Use hope as a driving force to advocate for policies and practices that promote social and political plurality. Encourage individuals to engage with their elected representatives, attend public meetings, or participate in peaceful protests to make their voices heard.

7. Lead by example: Embody the values of hope, inclusivity, and respect in your own actions and interactions. Be a role model by actively seeking out diverse perspectives, practicing empathy, and promoting dialogue. Encourage others to do the same.

Remember, promoting social and political plurality requires long-term commitment and effort. By utilizing hope as a catalyst, you can inspire individuals and communities to work towards a more inclusive and diverse society.

Hope and social justice are deeply interconnected. Hope serves as a powerful catalyst for social justice movements, providing the motivation and inspiration needed to drive change. Here are some ways in which hope, and social justice are linked:

1. Inspiring action: Hope fuels the belief that positive change is possible, even in the face of adversity. It gives individuals and communities the courage to take action, advocate for justice, and work towards creating a fair and equitable society.

2. Motivating resilience: The pursuit of social justice often involves challenging existing power structures and advocating for marginalized groups. In the face of obstacles and setbacks, hope provides the resilience needed to persevere and continue fighting for justice.

3. Fostering solidarity: Hope could bring people together. It encourages individuals from diverse backgrounds to unite in the pursuit of a common goal, creating a sense of solidarity and collective action. When people come together with hope, they can amplify their voices and effect meaningful change.

4. Challenging systemic injustices: Hope challenges the status quo by highlighting the possibility of a more just and equitable society. It pushes individuals to question and challenge the systemic injustices that perpetuate inequality, discrimination, and oppression.

5. Promoting empathy and understanding: Hope encourages individuals to see beyond their own experiences and empathize with the struggles of others. It fosters a sense of compassion and understanding, promoting the values of equality and justice.

6. Amplifying marginalized voices: Hope gives voice to those who have been

historically marginalized and oppressed. It empowers individuals and communities to speak up, share their stories, and demand justice. Hope serves as a catalyst for social change by amplifying marginalized voices and creating space for their perspectives to be heard.

7. Building a better future: Hope envisions a future where social justice is the norm. It inspires individuals to work towards dismantling oppressive systems and creating a society that values equality, fairness, and dignity for all.

8. In summary, hope and social justice are intertwined. Hope inspires action, fosters resilience, and promotes solidarity in the pursuit of a more just and equitable world. It is an essential ingredient in the fight for social justice and the creation of a better future for all.

Hope, Justice, Plurality, Triangle of Leadership and Success:

Plurality, or recognizing and embracing diversity in all its forms, is closely linked to social justice. Here are some ways in which plurality and social justice intersect:

1. Inclusion and equity: Plurality acknowledges and values the diverse identities, backgrounds, and experiences of individuals and communities. Social justice aims to ensure that everyone has equal opportunities, rights, and access to resources. Embracing plurality is essential for creating inclusive and equitable societies where everyone's needs are met and their voices are heard.

2. Intersectionality: Plurality recognizes that individuals have multiple intersecting identities and experiences that shape their lives. Social justice recognizes the importance of considering these intersections and addressing the unique challenges faced by individuals who belong to multiple marginalized groups. Understanding and respecting these diverse identities is crucial for achieving justice and equality for all.

3. Representation and participation: Plurality promotes the representation and participation of diverse groups in decision-making processes and institutions. Social justice seeks to challenge power imbalances and ensure that marginalized

voices are included and empowered. Embracing plurality means actively creating spaces for people from different backgrounds to have a say in shaping policies and practices that affect their lives.

4. Addressing systemic oppression: Plurality acknowledges that systemic oppression exists and affects different groups in different ways. Social justice aims to dismantle these oppressive systems and structures and create a more just society. Recognizing and understanding the diverse experiences of marginalized groups is crucial for identifying and addressing the root causes of injustice and working towards systemic change.
5. Cultivating empathy and understanding: Plurality encourages individuals to recognize and appreciate different perspectives and experiences. Social justice seeks to challenge prejudice, discrimination, and stereotypes. Embracing plurality allows us to cultivate empathy, understanding, and respect for others, fostering a more inclusive and compassionate society.
6. Celebrating diversity: Plurality embraces the richness and beauty of human diversity. Social justice recognizes the inherent worth and dignity of all individuals, regardless of their backgrounds. By celebrating and valuing diversity, we can challenge social norms, promote acceptance, and create environments where everyone can thrive.

In summary, hope and social justice are intertwined. Hope inspires action, fosters resilience, and promotes solidarity in the pursuit of a more just and equitable world. It is an essential ingredient in the fight for social justice and the creation of a better future for all. plurality and social justice are intertwined. Embracing plurality is essential for achieving social justice, as it involves recognizing and addressing the diverse needs, experiences, and identities of individuals and communities. By working towards a more inclusive and equitable society, we can create a world where everyone could live with dignity and justice.

INCORPORATING HOPE IN FIGHTING DICTATORSHIP

Promoting and advancing hope, plurality, and social justice in an ideological dictatorship system can be challenging, but there are still actions that individuals and communities can take to make a difference. Here are some strategies that can be helpful:

1- Raise awareness: Educate yourself and others about the concepts of hope, plurality, and social justice. Share information and engage in discussions to create awareness about the importance of these values. Use different platforms, such as social media, community gatherings, or local publications, to reach a wider audience.

2- Build alliances: Identify like-minded individuals and organizations who are also committed to promoting hope, plurality, and social justice. Collaborate with them to create a stronger collective voice. By working together, you can amplify your efforts and create a network of support.

3- Engage in peaceful resistance: Peacefully resist oppressive policies and actions by participating in protests, demonstrations, or advocacy campaigns. Use creative and nonviolent methods to express your dissent and draw attention to injustices. This can help raise public awareness and put pressure on the regime to address social justice concerns.

4- Support local initiatives: Identify and support grassroots initiatives that aim to promote social justice and plurality. This could involve volunteering, providing resources, or fundraising for organizations that work towards these goals. By supporting local initiatives, you can contribute to positive change at a community level.

5- Foster dialogue and empathy: Encourage open and respectful dialogue among individuals with different perspectives. Seek common ground and engage in conversations that foster understanding and empathy. By promoting dialogue, you can challenge the divide created by the dictatorship and create spaces for diverse voices to be heard.

6- Utilize technology and media: Use technology and media platforms to share stories, experiences, and information related to hope, plurality, and social justice. Utilize social media, online blogs, or independent media outlets to amplify marginalized voices, challenge propaganda, and promote alternative narratives.

International advocacy: Seek support from international human rights organizations, NGOs, or international bodies that specialize in promoting human rights and social justice. Engage with them to raise awareness about the situation in the dictatorship and advocate for international pressure to address human rights abuses.

Cultivate hope and resilience: Foster a sense of hope and resilience within yourself and your community. Encourage people to hold onto their dreams for a better future, despite the challenges they may face. Support each other emotionally and provide spaces for healing and self-care.

Remember that promoting hope, plurality, and social justice in an ideological dictatorship system can be risky, so it's important to prioritize personal safety and consider the context in which you are working. Adapt your strategies based on the specific circumstances and always prioritize the well-being of yourself and others involved.

Forgotten Country, Iran

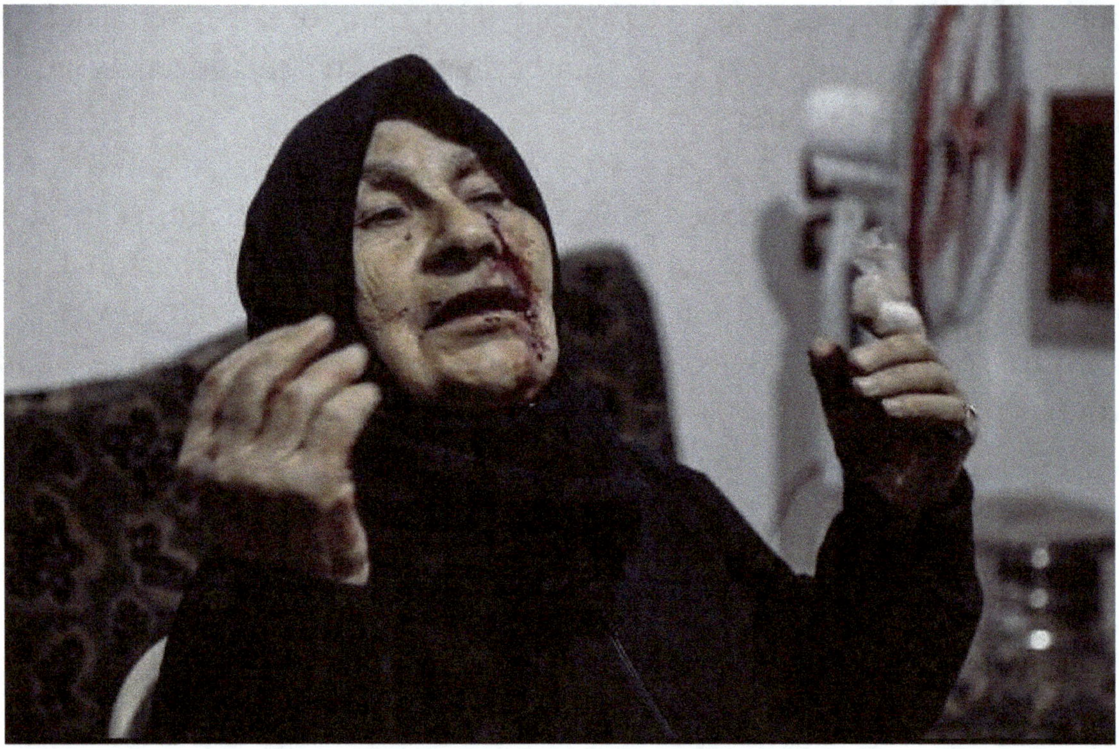

Current State of health care

First Steps, A Road Map to Immediate Accessibility and Care Assess, Verify and Utilize general information about healthcare deficiencies that exist in Iran:

Healthcare deficiencies can vary and may include issues such as limited access to healthcare services, inadequate infrastructure, a shortage of healthcare professionals, insufficient funding, unequal distribution of resources, and challenges in providing quality care to all segments of the population. It's always important to refer to reliable sources or news outlets for the most up-to- date information on healthcare deficiencies in Iran. Unfortunately, many information, news and representations from Iran are engineered, fabricatedand far from truth.

Key Points:

1. Access to Healthcare: lack of access to healthcare services, such as limited healthcare facilities, healthcare professionals, and medical equipment.
2. Quality of Care: Substandard quality of healthcare services, including inadequate infrastructure, outdated medical technology, and shortages of essential medical

supplies.

3. Health Disparities: Inequalities in healthcare, such as disparities based on income, rural-urban divide, and marginalized populations facing additional barriers to healthcare access.
4. Chronic Disease Burden: Rising burden of chronic diseases, such as diabetes, cardiovascular diseases, and respiratory conditions, malnutrition and the need for effective prevention and management strategies.
5. Maternal and Child Health: One of the major issues of healthcare in Iran are the challenges in maternal and child health, including high maternal and infant mortality rates, limited access to prenatal and postnatal care, and inadequate nutrition for mothers and children.
6. Mental Health: Lack of mental health services and resources, high prevalence of mental health disorders and substance abuse, warrants immediate action and increased investment in mental healthcare.

Statistics:

1. Percentage of the population without access to healthcare services. Reported data, figures and statistics by Islamic republic and affiliated academics are unreelable.

2. Maternal and infant mortality rates despite current reports are in the rise.

3. Life expectancy and mortality rates for major diseases, the life expectancy is dropping to low 60s and chronic diseases such as cardiovascular diseases are ramping up.

4. Percentage of healthcare facilities with inadequate infrastructure or equipment, Iran reports 7% of total GPD on healthcare, but the data from Iran descents is less than 6% and around 4.5%.

Iran has less than 900 (954) hospitals and 3700 clinics, 60% state controlled.

Total number of hospitals in select countries worldwide in 2022	
Characteristic	**Number of hospitals**
Colombia	**10,899**
Japan	8,205
United States	6,129
Mexico	5,019

5. Number of healthcare professionals per capita, Iran reports about 134000 physicians in the country (actual number is 99000). Based on their report there are 1.5 physician per 1000 individuals.

Iran report 0.8 nurses (actual 0.5) per hospital bed (required recommendation is 2.5) .

6. Prevalence rates of chronic diseases and mental health disorders.

Cause	Men	Women
Stroke	31.2 (14.5-47.4)	16.9 (7.2-26.6)
Lower respiratory infection	32.5 (8.3-56.8)	49.8 (33.6-66.1)
Diabetes	19.1 (15.0-23.2)	36.9 (28.5-45.2)
Other	40.6 (34.3-46.9)	39.8 (32.5-47.0)

Islamic Republic of Iran has one of the highest age standardized prevalence rates of cardiovascular diseases in the world, more than 9000 cases per 100 000 people. Global age -standardized cardiovascular death in 2022 was 553 per 100 000

Cause of death	Frequency		
	Male	Female	Total
Cardiovascular diseases	65	30	95
Motor vehicle accidents	52	12	64
Cancers	25	16	41
Unintentional injuries	14	9	23
Intentional injuries	20	2	22
Stroke	8	2	10
Lower respiratory infections	5	3	8
Diabetes	4	2	6
Other	48	43	91
Total	241	119	360

Recommendations:

1. Increase or reallocate healthcare funding: Advocate for increased investment in healthcare infrastructure (intermediate), medical equipment, and healthcare workforce.
2. Improve healthcare access: In addition to utilizing existing services, develop and implement policies to improve access to healthcare services, particularly in underserved areas.
3. Enhance medical education and training: Strengthen medical education programs to produce more healthcare professionals and improve the quality of healthcare services.
4. Preventive care: Promote preventive healthcare measures to reduce the burden of chronic diseases and improve overall population health.
5. Health disparities: Implement targeted interventions to address health disparities based on income, geography, and marginalized populations.
6. Prioritize mental health: Allocate resources to improve mental healthcare services and raise awareness about mental health issues.

Understanding the Healthcare and Shortages:

"Lack of quantity leads to a lack of quality"

1. Access to Healthcare Predictors of Good Health and Well-Being of a Nation:

- Percentage of the population without access to healthcare services.

- Number of healthcare facilities per capita.

- Distance and travel time to the nearest healthcare facility. - Availability of healthcare professionals, such as doctors and nurses.

> Global healthcare guidelines suggest a nurse-to-patient ratio of approximately 2.5 for optimal care. However, Iran has only **0.8 nurses available for each hospital bed**. Oct 24, 2023

2. Quality of Care Indicators:

- Mortality rates for major diseases, such as cardiovascular diseases, cancer, or infectious diseases.

- Patient satisfaction ratings with healthcare services.

- Availability of essential medical equipment and technology.

- Rates of healthcare-associated infections.

3. Health Disparities:

- Disparities in healthcare access and outcomes based on income, education, or geographic location.

- Maternal and infant mortality rates among different population groups.

- Differences in life expectancy between various demographic groups.

4. Chronic Disease Burden:

- Prevalence rates of major chronic diseases, such as diabetes, hypertension, or respiratory conditions.

- Rates of hospitalization or emergency room visits due to chronic diseases.

- Availability and utilization of preventive healthcare services, such as screenings and vaccinations.

> A cohort-based study in Iran (2013), showed that CVDs mortality rate in men and women was 331 and 203 per 100,000 people per year, which is almost two times higher than the average income of countries [39]. These pieces of evidence

Cause	Men	Women
Stroke	31.2 (14.5-47.4)	16.9 (7.2-26.6)
Lower respiratory infection	32.5 (8.3-56.8)	49.8 (33.6-66.1)
Diabetes	19.1 (15.0-23.2)	36.9 (28.5-45.2)
Other	40.6 (34.3-46.9)	39.8 (32.5-47.0)

5. Maternal and Child Health:

- Maternal mortality rates.

- Infant mortality rates.

- Rates of prenatal and postnatal care utilization.

- Malnutrition rates among children.

6. Mental Health:

Iran has the highest age-standardized rate of mental health disorders ahead of Australia and New Zealand (WHO)

- Prevalence rates of mental health disorders in the population.

The prevalence of psychiatric disorders was 10.81%. It was more common among females than males (14.34% vs. 7.34%, $P < 0.001$). The prevalence of anxiety and mood disorders were 8.35% and 4.29% respectively. The prevalence of psychotic disorders was 0.89%; neuro-cognitive disorders, 2.78% and dissociative disorders, 0.77%. Among mood disorders, major depressive disorder (2.98%) and among anxiety disorders, phobic disorder (2.05%) had the higher prevalence. The prevalence of psychiatric disorders among divorced and separated 22.31%; residents of urban areas 11.77%; illiterates 13.80%; householders 15.48%; unemployed 12.33% that were more than other groups.

ClinPrac Epidmiol Ment Health 2005

- Availability and accessibility of mental healthcare services.
- Rates of suicide or self-harm.

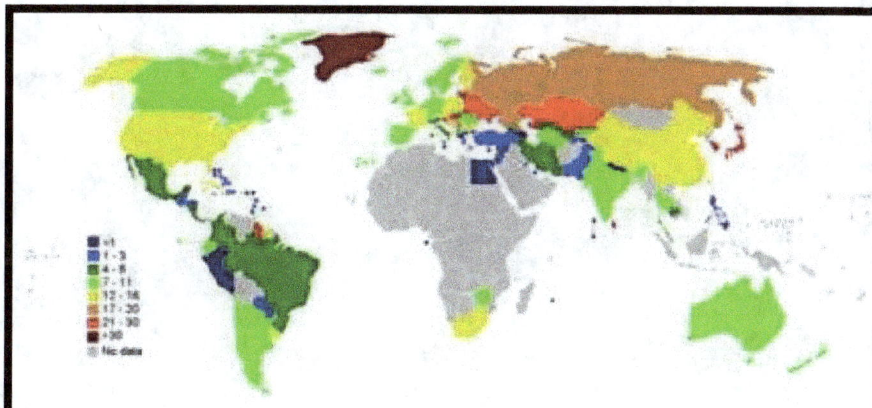

Iran's suicide rate per 100,000 people compared to other countries, according to the World Health Organization, Geneva. Peeter Värnik in 2012.[1]

Alarming Rate of Suicides in Iran in 2023: A Consequence of the Religious Dictatorship

By **IranNewsW2** — 12 months Ago

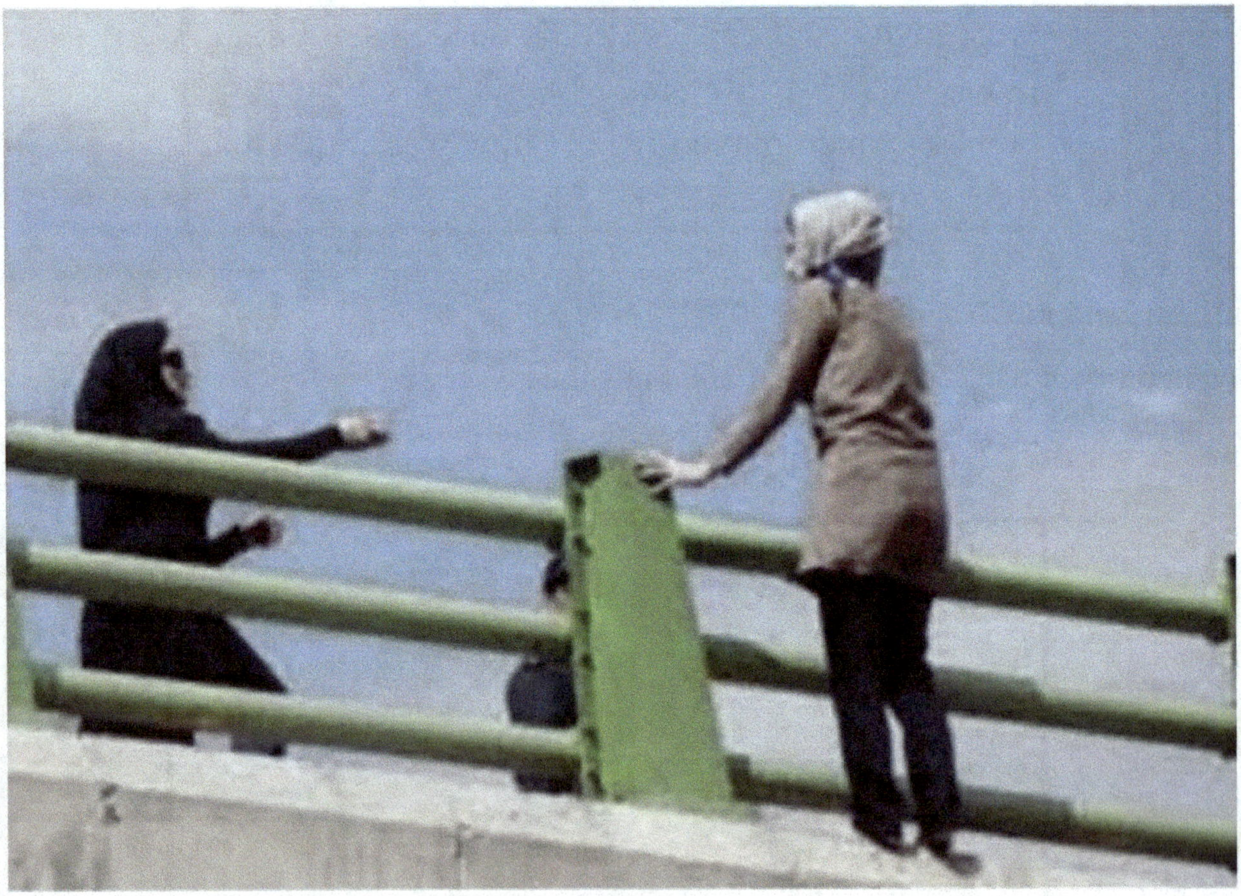

Archive

Increase in Suicide Rate Over the Last Two Decades

According to the Sociological Association of Iran, presented statistics on the suicide rate in Iran show that, in the last two decades, the suicide rate in the country has increased by 44%.

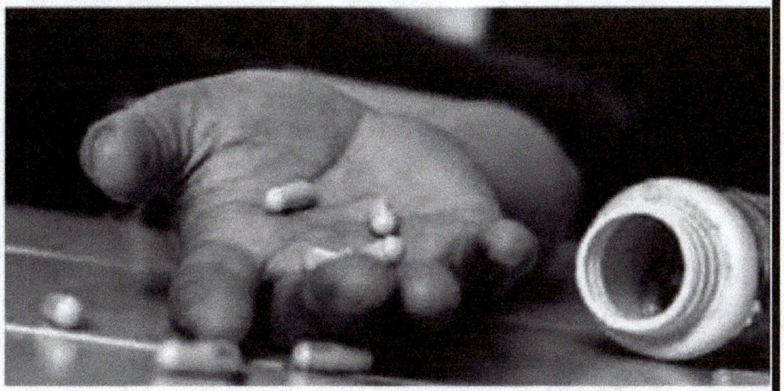

Several factors contribute to the quality of care in a healthcare system:

1. Healthcare Professionals:

- Competence and expertise of healthcare providers, including doctors, nurses, and specialists.
- Continuous education and professional development opportunities for healthcare professionals.
- Adequate staffing levels to ensure patient safety and minimize workload burden.

The NEW ENGLAND JOURNAL of MEDICINE

REVIEW ARTICLE | GLOBAL HEALTH

Global Supply of Health Professionals

FIGURE 1

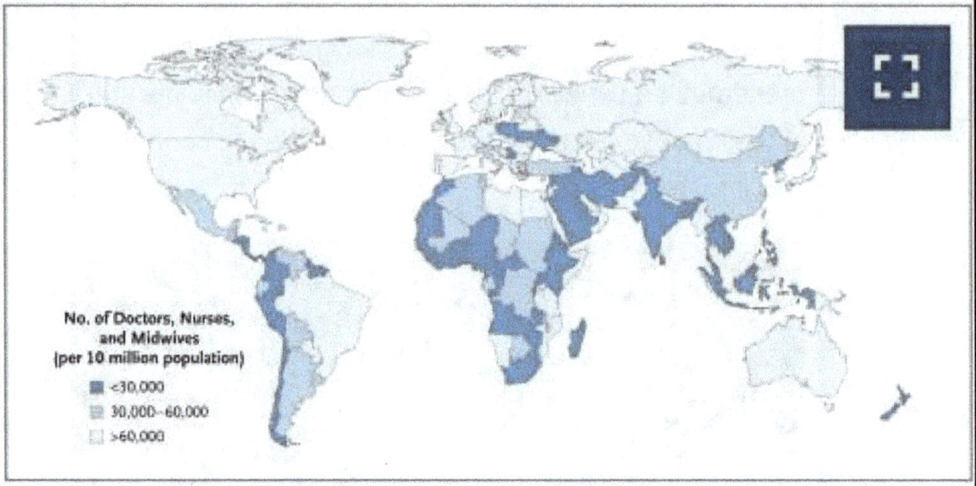

Doctors, Nurses, and Midwives per 10 Million Population, 2011.

FIGURE 2

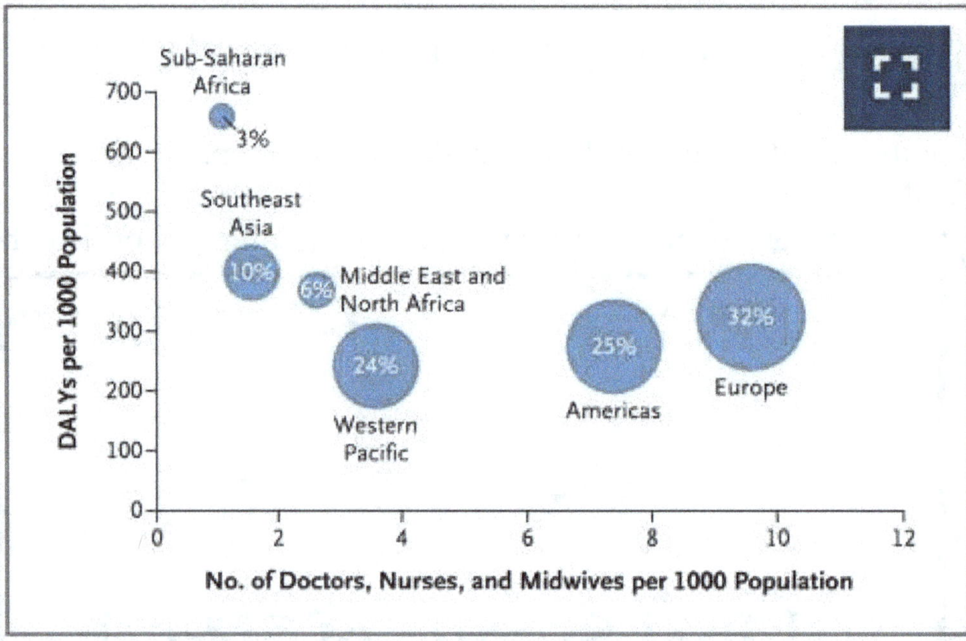

Global Health Workforce and Burden of Disease According to WHO Region.

2. Access to Healthcare:

- Availability and accessibility of healthcare services, including primary care, specialized care, and emergency services.

- **Timely access to appointments, diagnostic tests, and treatments.**

Iran Under the Rule of the Islamic Republic

- Culture and History. Iran prior to the Islamic Republic was rich in its culture and history.
- Creation of "Supreme Leader" ...
- Human Rights Abuses. ...
- Support for Terrorism. ...
- Iran's Missile Program. ...
- Illicit Financial Activities. ...
- Threat to Maritime Security. ...
- Environmental Exploitation.

- Affordability of healthcare services, including insurance coverage and out-of-packet costs

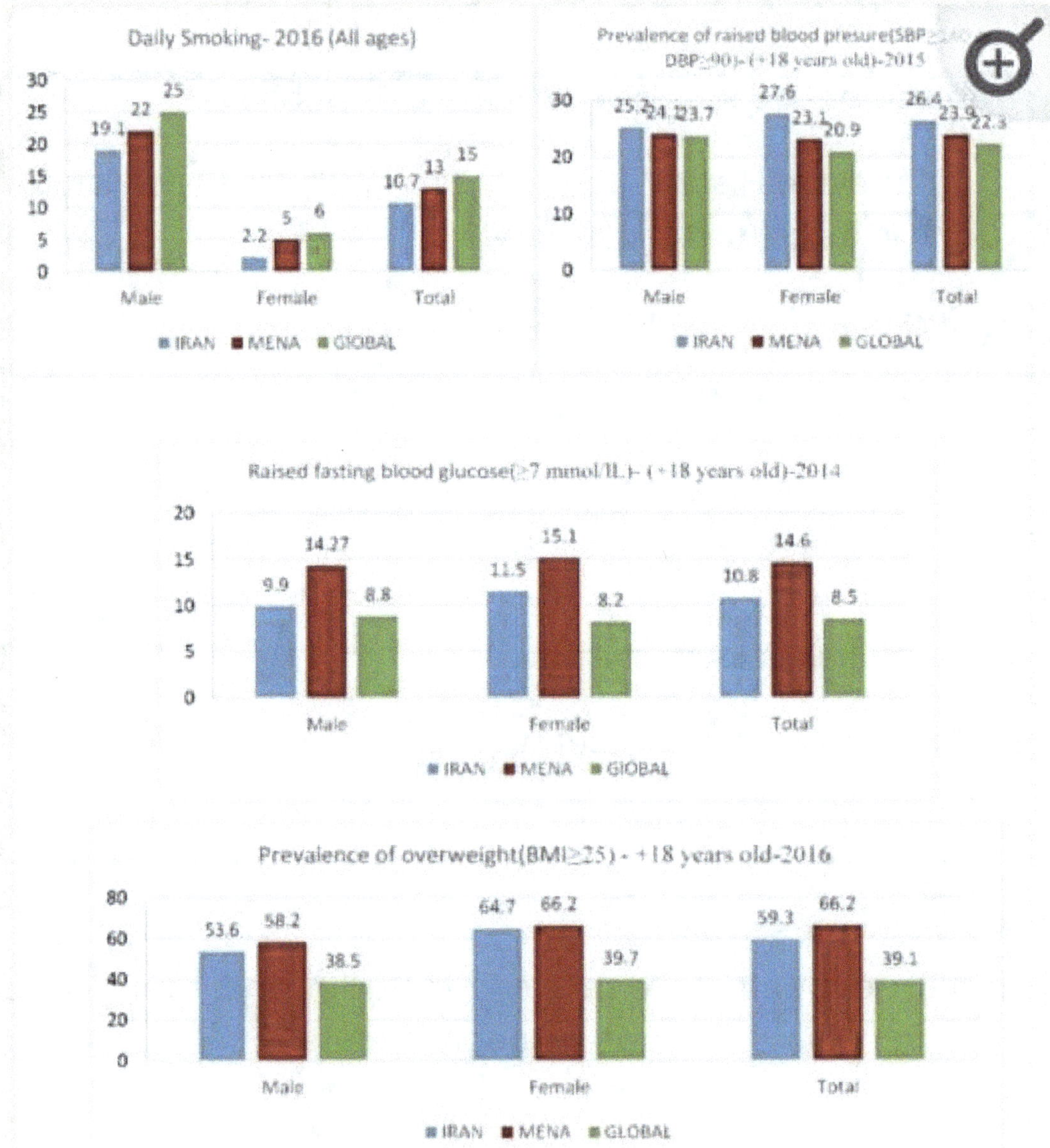

Fig. 3:

Prevalence of NCDs risk factors in Iran, MENA and the world (last available data)

According to the government of Iran, **about 60 percent of Iranians are overweight and 35 percent of women and 15 percent of men suffer from obesity in Iran**. Despite the young age of many Iranians, only 20 percent of Iranians are physically active while the world average is 60 percent.

W https://en.m.wikipedia.org › wiki

Health in Iran - Wikipedia

PHC system of Iran is facing the problem of shortage of funds for its programs, some issues such as; **inefficient health systems and high administrative costs** had been highlighted this problem (28). A variety of health service financing systems was expressed as important challenge for PHC system of Iran (29).

After random effect model meta-analysis, the questionnaire-based prevalence of food insecurity in the Iran was 49.2% (without hunger 29.6% and with hunger 19.2%). In other words, **less than half of the households are facing with food insecurity**.

https://www.ncbi.nlm.nih.gov › pmc

Frequency distribution and Gini coefficient of active physicians by specialty in Iran in 2019

Ophthalmology	1707	2.14	Bushehr
Nose and Throat and Head and Neck Surgery	1314	1.64	Sistan and Baluchestan
Neurosurgery	615	0.77	Sistan and Baluchestan
Dermatology	1032	1.29	Sistan and Baluchestan
Radiotherapy	257	0.32	Semnan
Nuclear medicine	180	0.23	Kohgiloyeh and Boyerahmad
Physical medicine and rehabilitation	348	0.44	Ilam
Forensic Medicine	252	0.32	Kohgiloyeh and Boyerahmad
Occupational Medicine	141	0.18	-
Sports medicine	65	0.08	-
Geriatrics	10	0.01	-

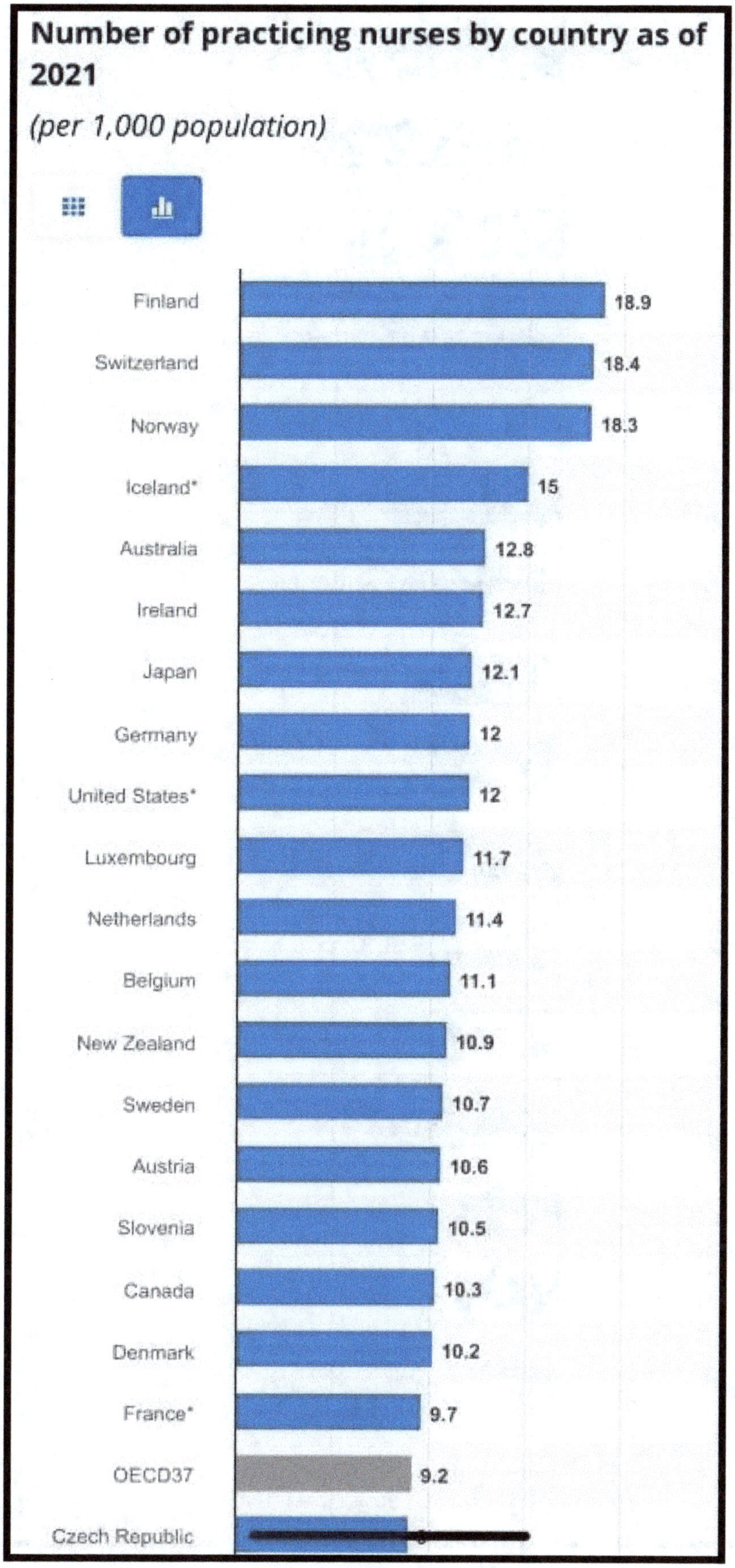
Number of practicing nurses by country as of 2021
(per 1,000 population)
Finland
18.9
Switzerland
18.4
Norway
18.3
Iceland*
15
Australia
12.8
Ireland
12.7
Japan
12.1
Germany
12
United States*
12
Luxembourg
11.7
Netherlands
11.4
Belgium
11.1
New Zealand
10.9
Sweden
10.7
Austria
10.6
Slovenia
10.5
Canada
10.3
Denmark
10.2
France*
9.7
OECD37
9.2
Czech Republic

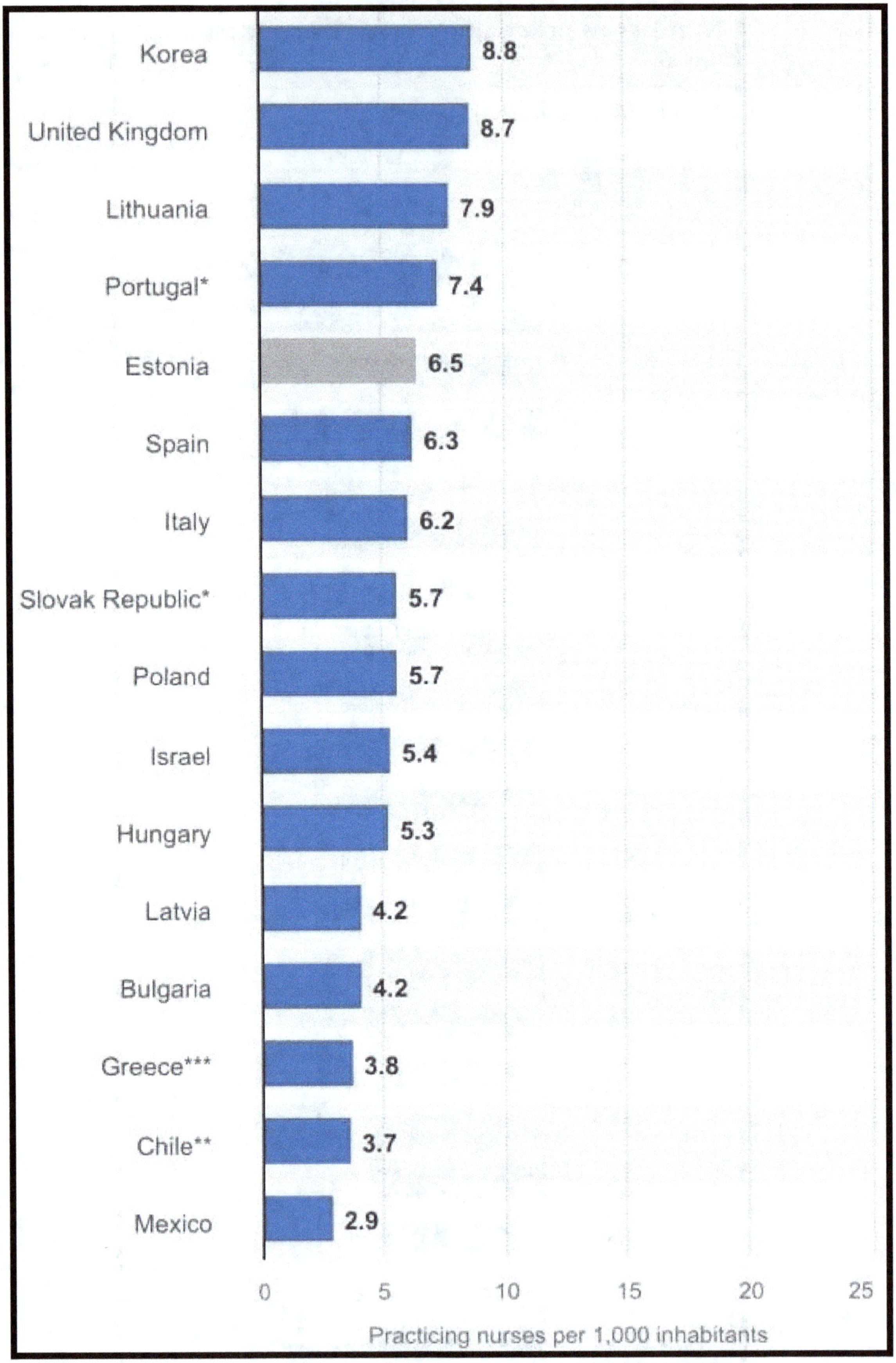

Korea
8.8
United Kingdom
8.7
Lithuania
7.9
Portugal*
7.4
Estonia
6.5
Spain
6.3
Italy
6.2
Slovak Republic*
5.7
Poland
5.7
Israel
5.4
Hungary
5.3
Latvia
4.2
Bulgaria
4.2
Greece***
3.8
Chile**
3.7
Mexico
2.9
0
5
10
15
20
25
Practicing nurses per 1,000 inhabitants

The distribution of active physicians in different provinces of the country was shown in Figure 2. Most of the provinces had 20–40 specialist physicians per 100,000 population.

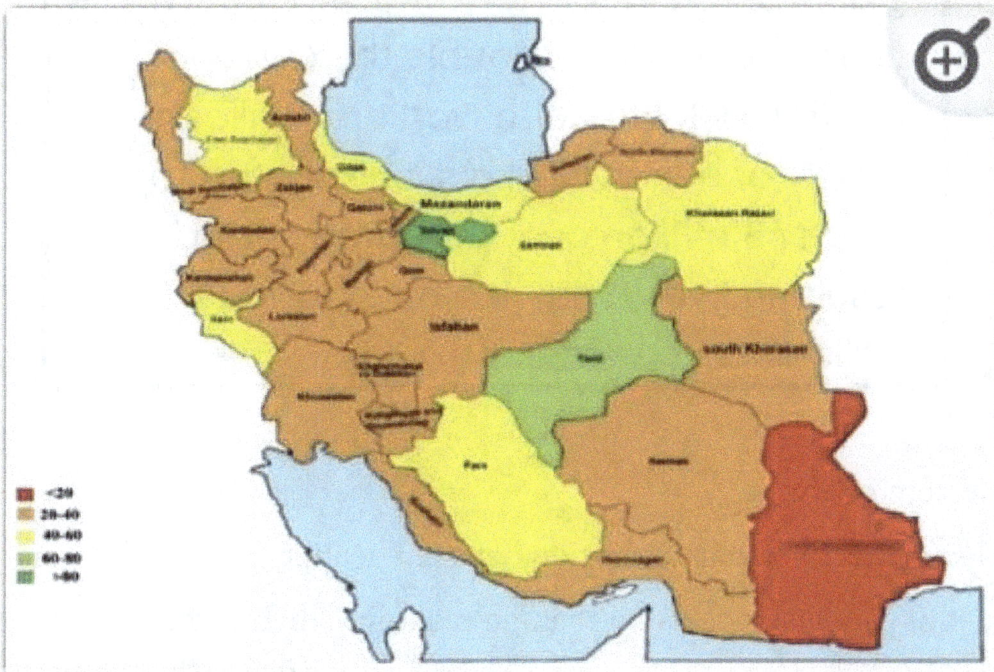

Figure 2

The distribution of active specialist physicians in different Iranian provinces in 2019

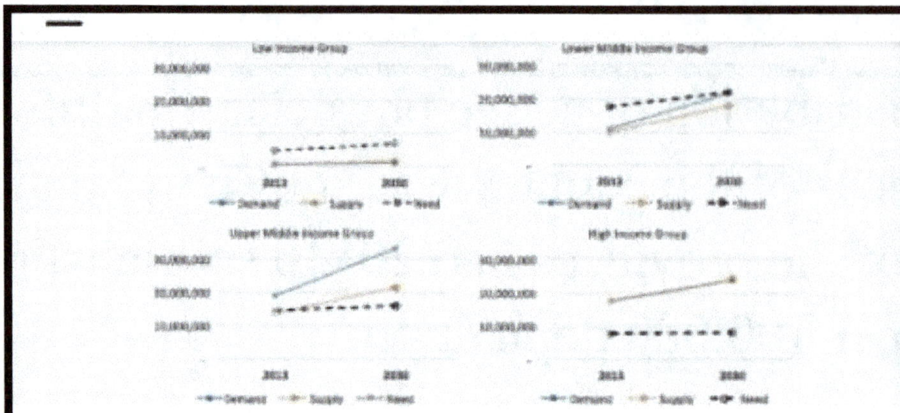

Results. The model predicts that, by 2030, global demand for health workers will rise to 80 million workers, double the current (2013) stock of health workers, while the supply of health workers is expected to reach 65 million over the same period, resulting in a worldwide net shortage of 15 million health workers. Feb 3, 2017

3. Patient-Centered Care:

- Respectful and effective communication between healthcare providers and patients.
- Involvement of patients in decision-making regarding their healthcare.
- Coordination and continuity of care across different healthcare settings.

4. Evidence-Based Practice:

- Use of the latest research and best available evidence to guide clinical decision-making.
- Implementation of clinical guidelines and protocols.
- Monitoring and evaluation of healthcare outcomes to drive quality improvement initiatives.

5. Healthcare Infrastructure:

- Availability of essential medical equipment, technology, and medications.
- Well-maintained healthcare facilities with adequate resources.
- Effective information systems for patient records and healthcare.

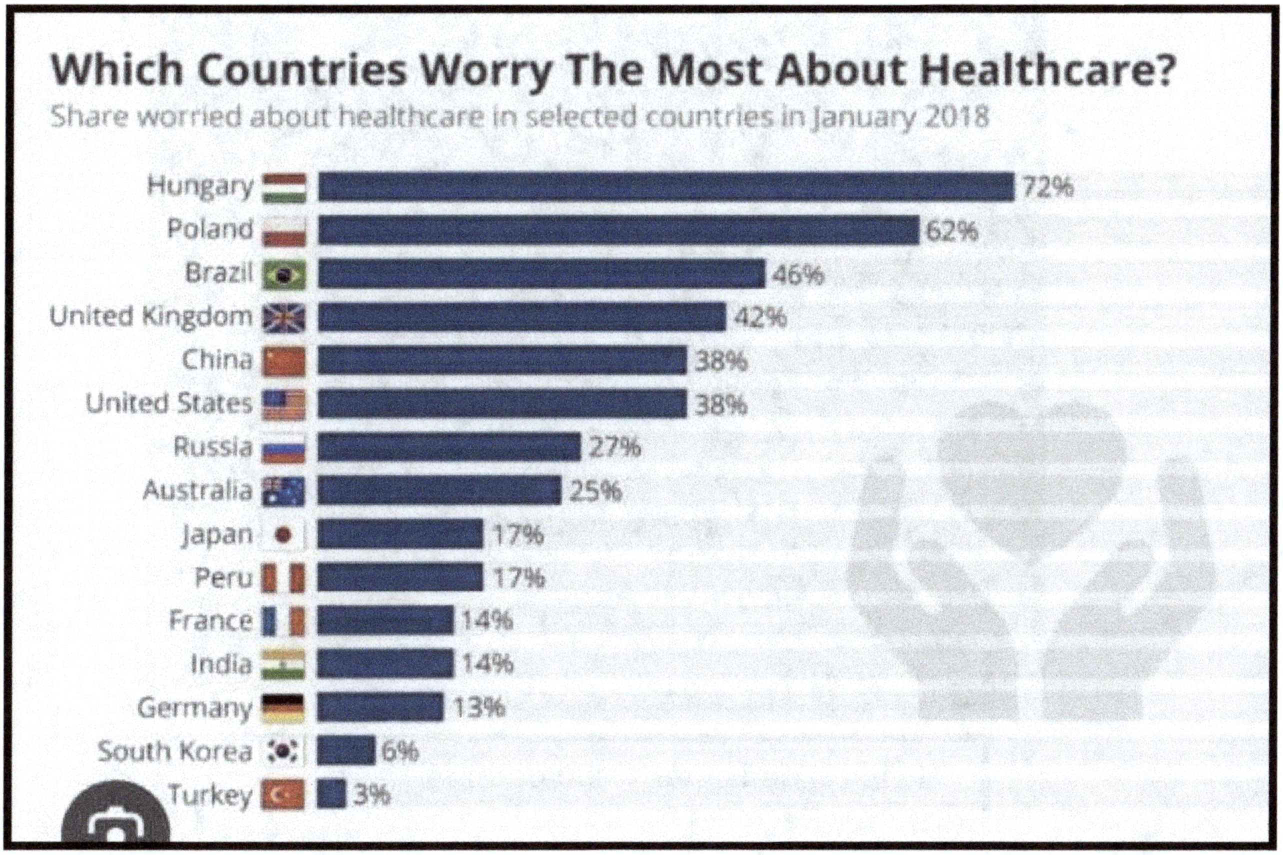

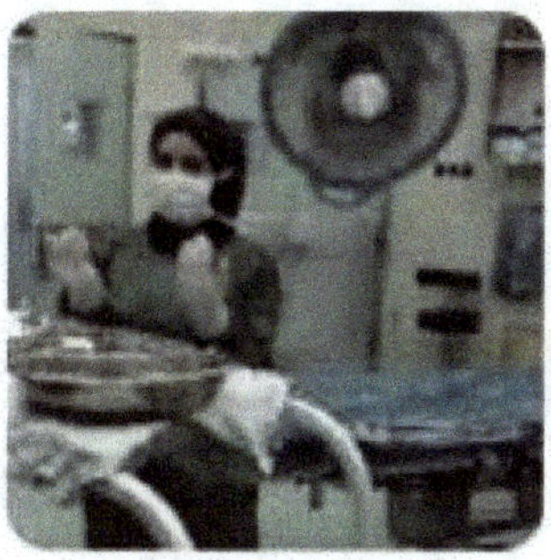

Iran spends about 7% of its GDP each year on health services and has an estimated **954 hospitals**, 3,700 clinics and 6,400 rehabilitation centers. About 60% of Iran's hospitals are state controlled with the remainder run by private companies or non-governmental organizations, including charities. Aug 8, 2018

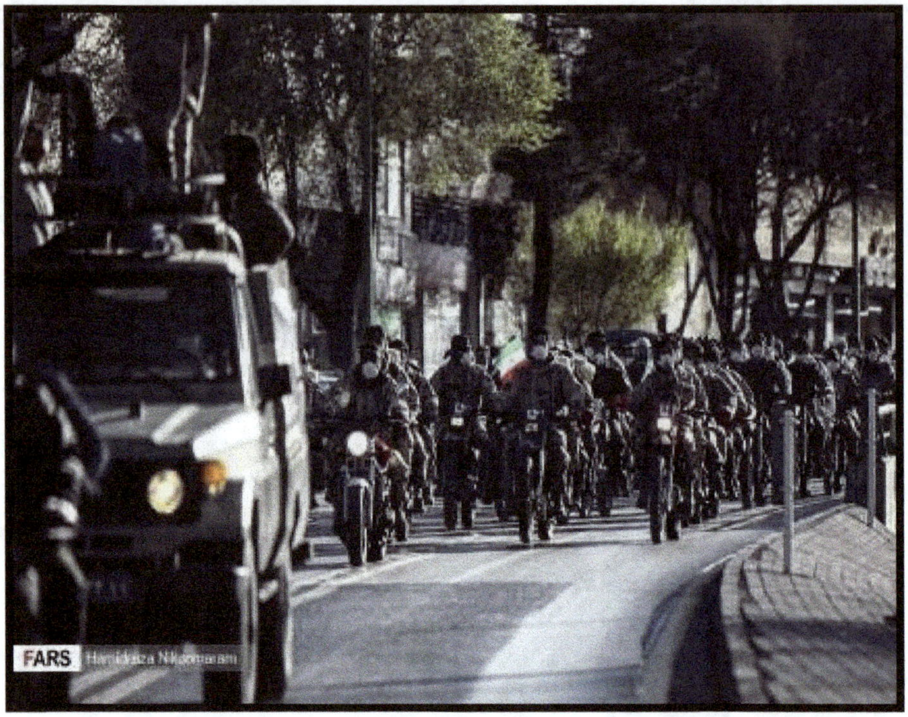
FARS

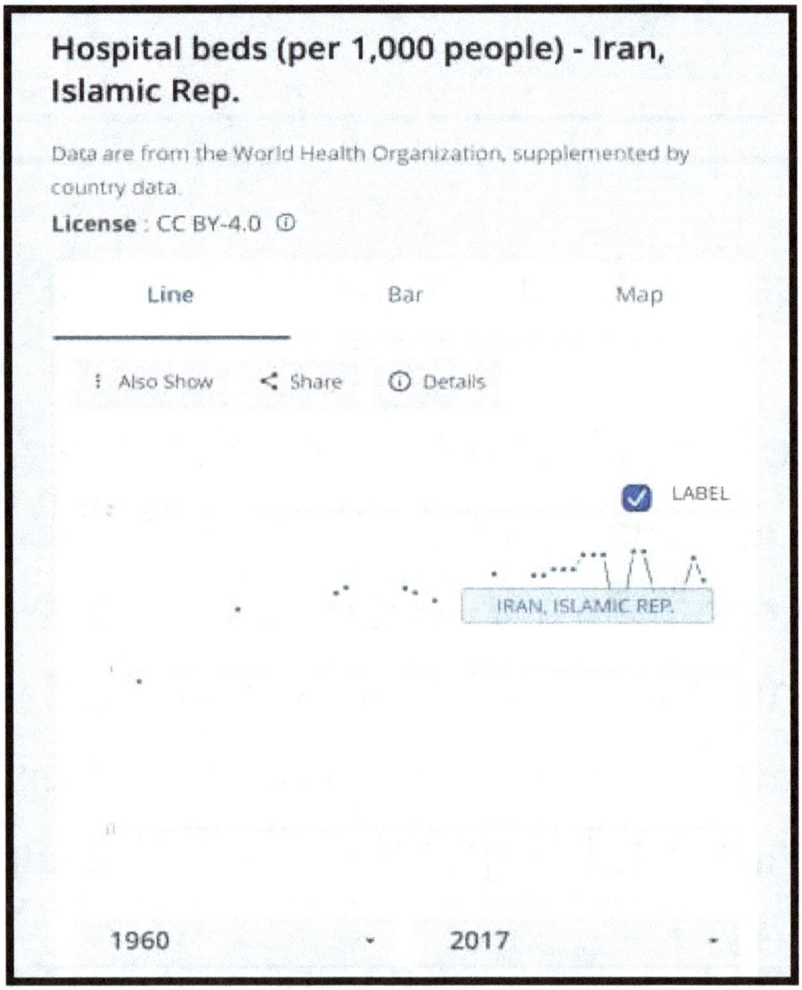
Hospital beds (per 1,000 people) - Iran, Islamic Rep.
Data are from the World Health Organization, supplemented by country data.
License : CC BY-4.0
Line
Bar
Map
Also Show
Share
Details
LABEL
IRAN, ISLAMIC REP.
1960
2017

Data

The distribution of active physicians in different provinces of the country was shown in Figure 2. Most of the provinces had 20–40 specialist physicians per 100,000 population.

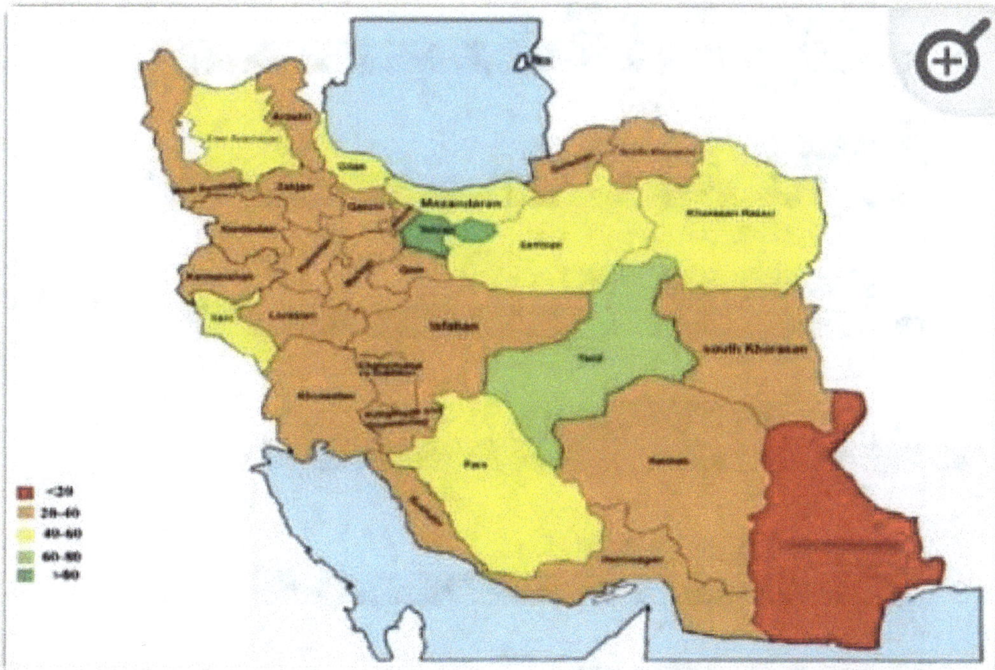

Figure 2

The distribution of active specialist physicians in different Iranian provinces in 2019

Management.

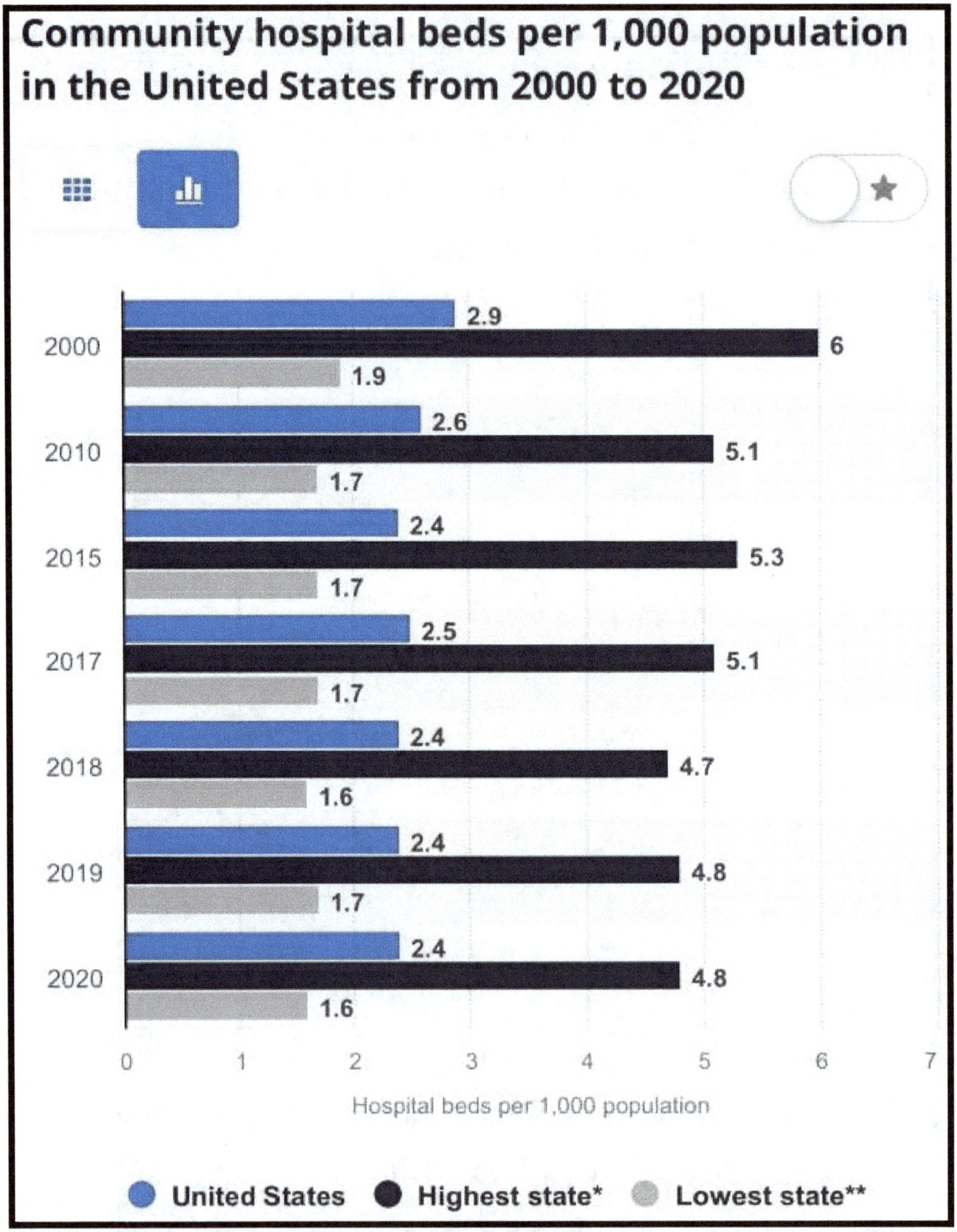
Community hospital beds per 1,000 population in the United States from 2000 to 2020
2000
2010
2015
2017
2018
2019
2020
2.9
6
1.9
2.6
5.1
1.7
2.4
5.3
1.7
2.5
5.1
1.7
2.4
4.7
1.6
2.4
4.8
1.7
2.4
4.8
1.6
0 1 2 3 4 5 6 7
Hospital beds per 1,000 population
United States
Highest state*
Lowest state**

Total number of hospitals in select countries worldwide in 2022

Characteristic	Number of hospitals
Colombia	**10,899**
Japan	8,205
United States	6,129
Mexico	5,019

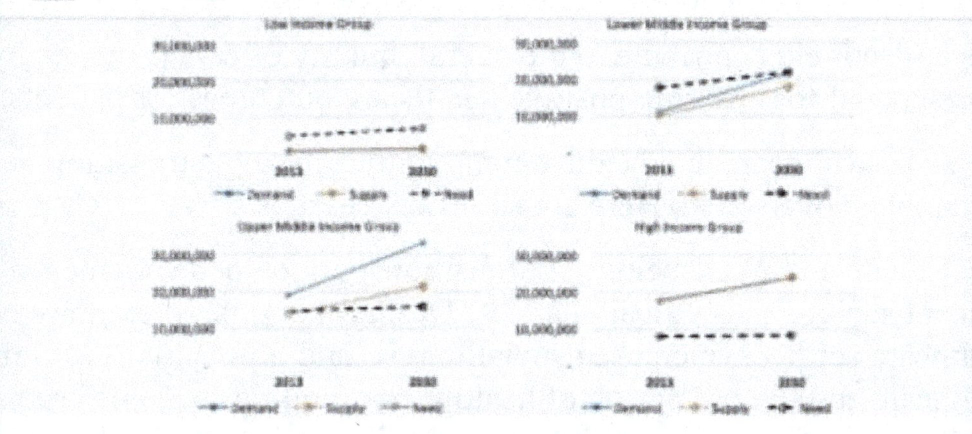

Results. The model predicts that, by 2030, global demand for health workers will rise to 80 million workers, double the current (2013) stock of health workers, while the supply of health workers is expected to reach **65 million** over the same period, resulting in a worldwide net shortage of 15 million health workers. Feb 3, 2017

6. Patient Safety:

- Implementation of protocols and practices to prevent medical errors and adverse events.

- Infection control measures to minimize healthcare-associated infections.

- Reporting and learning systems to identify and address patient safety incidents.

7. Health Information Systems:

- Efficient and secure electronic health records systems.

- Interoperability of health information systems to facilitate seamless exchange of patient information.

- Use of health data analytics to monitor and improve healthcare outcomes.

8. Continuous Quality Improvement:

- Regular monitoring and measurement of healthcare performance indicators.

- Feedback mechanisms for patients to report their experiences and provide input.

- Implementation of quality improvement initiatives based on data-driven insights.

These factors collectively contribute to the overall quality of care provided by a healthcare system and are crucial for ensuring positive healthcare outcomes for patients.

The importance of healthcare and healthy communities during a transition period to democracy cannot be overstated. Here are some key reasons why:

1. Public Health and Well-being: A transition period to democracy often involves significant social and political changes. During this time, there may be disruptions in healthcare services, increased social unrest, and a potential for violence. Access to healthcare and the promotion of healthy communities become crucial in ensuring the well-being of individuals and communities. Adequate healthcare services can prevent and address health issues that may arise during this period.

2. Stability and Social Cohesion: Healthcare services and healthy communities contribute to stability and social cohesion during a transition to democracy. By ensuring access to healthcare, promoting preventive measures, and addressing health disparities, communities can experience improved health outcomes. This fosters a sense of well-being, trust, and unity among individuals, which is essential for a smooth transition and the establishment of a stable democratic society.

3. Rebuilding Trust: Transition periods are often characterized by mistrust and skepticism towards institutions and authorities. Strengthening healthcare systems and promoting healthy communities can help rebuild trust between the government and the people. By delivering quality healthcare services, addressing community

health needs, and actively involving the community in decision-making processes, trust can be restored, laying the foundation for a healthy democratic society.

4. Addressing Inequalities: Transition periods may exacerbate existing social and health inequalities. Access to healthcare and the presence of healthy communities can help address these inequalities by ensuring that marginalized groups have equal opportunities for healthcare services and health promotion. This promotes social justice and creates a more inclusive society where everyone has equal access to quality healthcare.

5. Prevention of Health Crises: Transition periods often come with unique challenges and potential health crises. Effective healthcare systems and healthy communities can play a crucial role in preventing and responding to these crises. By focusing on preventive measures, early detection, and effective healthcare planning, communities can be better prepared to address health emergencies and mitigate their impact on the transition process.

6. Human Rights and Democracy: Access to healthcare is a fundamental human right, and the promotion of healthy communities is closely linked to the principles of democracy. During a transition to democracy, it is essential to uphold human rights, including the right to health. By prioritizing healthcare and healthy communities, societies can demonstrate their commitment to democratic values and the well-being of their citizens.

In summary, healthcare and healthy communities are essential during a transition period to democracy. They contribute to public health, stability, social cohesion, trust-building, addressing inequalities, prevention of health crises, and upholding human rights. By investing in healthcare and promoting healthy communities, societies can navigate the challenges of the transition process and build a strong foundation for a healthy and democratic future.

Revitalizing a deficient existing healthcare system and hospitals during a transition period with a new government requires careful planning and strategic actions. Here are some steps that can be taken:

1. Assess the Current Situation: Begin by conducting a comprehensive assessment of the existing healthcare system and hospitals. This includes evaluating infrastructure, equipment, human resources, financial resources, and service delivery. Identify the key areas of deficiency and prioritize the most critical issues that need immediate attention.

2. Develop a Strategic Plan: Create a strategic plan that outlines the goals, objectives, and actions required to revitalize the healthcare system and hospitals. This plan should be based on a thorough analysis of the current situation and should address the identified deficiencies. Set realistic targets and timelines for achieving the desired outcomes.

3. Allocate Sufficient Resources: Adequate financial and human resources are essential for revitalizing healthcare systems and hospitals. Work with the new government to allocate sufficient funds and ensure that healthcare facilities have the necessary staffing, medical supplies, and equipment to provide quality care. Seek external funding and partnerships if needed.

4. Strengthen Governance and Accountability: Establish strong governance mechanisms to ensure transparency, accountability, and effective management of healthcare systems and hospitals. This includes implementing robust monitoring and evaluation systems, promoting ethical practices, and enforcing regulations and standards. Foster a culture of accountability among healthcare providers and administrators.

5. Improve Infrastructure and Equipment: Upgrade the infrastructure of healthcare facilities and ensure that they are well equipped to provide quality care. This may involve renovating existing buildings, expanding facilities, or constructing new hospitals in areas with limited access to healthcare. Invest in modern medical equipment and technology to enhance diagnostic and treatment capabilities.

6. Enhance Human Resources: Invest in training and capacity-building programs for healthcare professionals. Provide opportunities for continuous professional development and ensure that healthcare workers are equipped with the necessary skills and knowledge to deliver quality care. Address workforce shortages by recruiting and retaining qualified healthcare professionals.

7. Strengthen Primary Healthcare: Focus on strengthening primary healthcare services as the foundation of the healthcare system. Enhance access to primary care facilities, promote preventive healthcare, and implement community-based health programs. This will help alleviate the burden on hospitals and improve overall healthcare outcomes.

8. Engage Stakeholders and the Community: Foster collaboration and engagement with key stakeholders, including healthcare professionals, community leaders, civil society organizations, and the public. Seek their input and involvement in decision-making processes, policy formulation, and healthcare planning. Build trust and partnerships to ensure the sustainability of healthcare initiatives.

9. Emphasize Health Promotion and Disease Prevention: Prioritize health promotion and disease prevention strategies to reduce the burden of preventable diseases. Implement public health campaigns, educate the public on healthy lifestyles, and provide access to immunizations and screenings. Focus on addressing social determinants of health and addressing health disparities.

10. Monitor Progress and Adapt: Regularly monitor the progress of the revitalization efforts and make necessary adjustments based on feedback and evaluation. Continuously assess the impact of interventions and make data-driven decisions to

ensure the effectiveness of healthcare systems and hospitals. Adapt the strategic plan as needed to address emerging challenges and changing healthcare needs.

Revitalizing a deficient healthcare system and hospitals during a transition period requires a long-term commitment and collaboration among various stakeholders. By implementing these steps, the new government can work towards improving healthcare access, quality, and outcomes, ultimately benefiting the population and building a stronger healthcare system for the future.

Addressing a deficient healthcare system in a corrupt country requires innovative thinking and out-of-the-box solutions. While there is no one-size-fits-all approach, here is an immediate solution that could help remedy the situation:

Establish a mobile healthcare initiative:

1. Mobile Clinics: Set up mobile clinics equipped with basic medical equipment and staffed by healthcare professionals. These clinics can travel to underserved areas, reaching remote communities that lack access to healthcare facilities. The clinics can provide primary healthcare services, including general check-ups, vaccinations, basic treatments, and health education.
2. Telemedicine: Utilize technology to provide remote medical consultations. Develop a telemedicine platform that allows patients to connect with healthcare professionals through video calls or chat. This can help overcome geographical barriers and allow individuals to receive medical advice and prescriptions without physically visiting a healthcare facility.
3. Community Health Workers: Train and empower community health workers who can act as a bridge between the healthcare system and the local population. These workers can provide basic healthcare services, and health education, and help identify individuals in need of specialized care. They can also assist in navigating the corrupt system and advocating for patients' rights.
4. Transparent Medical Supply Chain: Implement a transparent and accountable system for procuring and distributing medical supplies. Utilize technology, such as blockchain, to track the entire supply chain, ensuring that medicines and equipment reach the intended recipients without being diverted or stolen. This can help mitigate corruption and ensure the availability of essential healthcare resources.
5. Public-Private Partnerships: Foster collaborations between the public sector, private healthcare providers, and non-profit organizations. Encourage private hospitals and clinics to allocate a portion of their resources and expertise to provide subsidized or free healthcare services to underprivileged communities. This can help alleviate the burden on the public healthcare system and improve access to quality care.
6. Health Education and Prevention: Prioritize health education and prevention programs to empower individuals to take charge of their health. Conduct

community workshops, awareness campaigns, and school programs to educate people about basic health practices, hygiene, and disease prevention. By focusing on prevention, the burden on the healthcare system can be reduced in the long run.

7. Anti-Corruption Measures: Implement strict anti-corruption measures within the healthcare system. This can include regular audits, whistleblower protection, and transparent processes for reporting and addressing corruption cases. Strengthening accountability and transparency can help restore trust in the healthcare system and ensure that resources are allocated efficiently.

It is important to acknowledge that these immediate solutions may not address all the underlying issues within a corrupt healthcare system. Long-term systemic reforms and sustained efforts are necessary to create lasting change. Additionally, the success of these initiatives depends on the commitment and collaboration of various stakeholders, including government entities, healthcare professionals, civil society organizations, and international partners.

The use of Artificial Intelligence (AI) can play a significant role in rebuilding a deficient healthcare system and transforming medical education in a country after a transition to a new government. Here are some ways AI can be utilized:

1. Data Analysis and Insights: AI can analyze large volumes of healthcare data to identify patterns, trends, and insights that can inform decision-making and policy development. This can help the new government understand the current state of the healthcare system, identify areas of improvement, and prioritize interventions.

2. Predictive Analytics: AI algorithms can be used to predict disease outbreaks, patient outcomes, and healthcare resource needs. This can assist in proactive planning, resource allocation, and early intervention strategies. By leveraging AI, the healthcare system can move from a reactive approach to a proactive one, leading to better health outcomes.

3. Telemedicine and Remote Care: AI-powered telemedicine platforms can enable remote consultations, diagnosis, and monitoring of patients, particularly in underserved areas. This can help bridge the gap between healthcare providers and patients, improving access to healthcare services and reducing the burden on physical infrastructure. AI algorithms can also assist in triaging patients and identifying those who require immediate medical attention.

4. Health Information Systems: AI can enhance the efficiency and accuracy of health information systems by automating tasks such as data entry, coding, and record management. This reduces the administrative burden on healthcare professionals, allowing them to focus more on patient care. AI can also facilitate interoperability

between different health information systems, enabling seamless data exchange and collaboration.

5. Medical Education and Training: AI technologies can revolutionize medical education by providing interactive and personalized learning experiences. Virtual reality (VR) and augmented reality (AR) simulations can be used to train medical students and healthcare professionals in a realistic and immersive environment. AI-powered virtual assistants can also provide on-demand access to medical knowledge and assist in clinical decision-making.

6. Clinical Decision Support: AI algorithms can analyze patient data, medical literature, and best practices to provide evidence-based recommendations to healthcare providers at the point of care. This can help improve diagnostic accuracy, treatment planning, and patient outcomes. AI-powered decision support systems can also assist in detecting medication errors, adverse drug reactions, and potential conflicts in treatment plans.

7. Resource Optimization: AI can optimize the allocation of healthcare resources, such as hospital beds, surgical facilities, and medical equipment. By analyzing data on patient flow, demand patterns, and resource availability, AI algorithms can help healthcare administrators make data-driven decisions to ensure efficient utilization of resources and reduce wait times.

8. Public Health Surveillance: AI can enhance public health surveillance by analyzing data from various sources, such as social media, wearable devices, and electronic health records. This can help identify emerging health threats, monitor population health indicators, and facilitate early intervention strategies. AI algorithms can also assist in contact tracing during disease outbreaks.

9. Ethical Considerations: The use of AI in healthcare should be guided by ethical considerations. Transparency, fairness, privacy, and accountability should be prioritized to ensure that AI systems are unbiased and secure and protect patient confidentiality. The new government should establish regulations and frameworks to govern the use of AI in healthcare and ensure its responsible and ethical implementation.

10. Collaboration and Partnerships: The new government should foster collaborations and partnerships with AI experts, technology companies, research institutions, and international organizations. This can facilitate knowledge transfer, access to AI expertise, and funding opportunities for AI initiatives in healthcare. Collaboration can also help address potential challenges and ensure that AI solutions are tailored to the specific needs and context of the country.

By harnessing the power of AI, the new government can rebuild a deficient healthcare system and transform medical education in the country. AI can improve healthcare access, quality, and efficiency, leading to better health outcomes for the population. However, it is crucial to ensure that AI is implemented responsibly, ethically, and in collaboration with relevant stakeholders to maximize its potential benefits.

Geriatric Health Overview

Geriatric care and the well-being of older Iranians are vastly ignored and underfunded.

One of the best models of care regardless of the geography is person-centered, holistic, and carefully individualized.

Person-centered care:
This involves recognizing the individuality of each older Iranian, their cultural views, region ethnic origin, and values.
Elder care is dynamic and it also involves actively engaging older individuals, their families, and caregivers. This process will ensure their dignity, privacy, and respect.
Holistic care: The care of older people is complex and involves a multi-disciplinary and team approach. This in addition to managing physical healthcare, also addresses mental, Emotional, and social well-being.

Coordination and integration of care:
This will guarantee seamless care across the healthcare system and different providers. This will be achieved by implementing care coordinators and care manager teams and And use of technology to facilitate communications and data sharing.

Preventive and early intervention:
This guarantees identifying and addressing health and disease issues early before They become more serious, which might need more intensive and costly interventions

Empowerment and self-management:
This involves ensures the involvement of older person to assume an active role in managing their health and well-being
This will be achieved through education, coaching, partnership with healthcare teams

Continuous quality improvement:
This will be achieved by regularly and closely monitoring reviewing and continuously improving the services that have been rendered.
This process will be achieved through partnership with healthcare teams, feedback by all parties involved, data analysis, and benchmarking against best practice models and Standards.

One of the best models of care for older people ie geriatric population as mentioned above is the "vertical model" of care based on a multidisciplinary team-based approach.

This will be structured as follows:

1. Multidisciplinary team-based care: professionals with different areas of expertise, geriatricians, nurses, pharmacists, social workers, physical therapists, and other providers as needed
2. Comprehensive geriatric assessment: a systemic evaluation of an older person's physical, mental, functional, cognitive, social, and psychological needs.
3. Coordination care: elder care is complex and somehow labor-intensive. Older care needs close and continuous coordination across the providers, hospitals, home, and community.
4. Continuity of care: since older individuals have more complex and multiple health issues and needs, therefore, elder care is ongoing and should be tailored to address changes in health and disease processes.
5. Patient-centered care: this will be achieved by directly involving the patient and family in decision-making and issues associated with end-of-life issues.
6. family and caregiver support: this is one of the most important components of elder care yet mostly underperformed or ignored.
7. It involves ongoing information sharing and education to familiarize the family with treatment plans and management strategies.

Islamic Republic of Iran

Medical Education and Professionalism Disparities, Failures, and Solutions

IR constitution defines the country as an Islamic republic and specifies Twelver Ja'afari Shai Islam as the official state religion. It states all laws and regulations must be based on Islamic Criteria and an official interpretation of Sharia.

The constitution states citizens shall enjoy human, political, economic, and other rights in conformity with Islamic Criteria.

The penal code provides for hudud punishments including amputation, flogging, and stoning (Iran 2022 International Religious Freedom Report).

Sharia law refers to the legal system based on the principles of Islamic religious teachings, primarily derived from the Quran and the Hadith (sayings and actions of Prophet Muhammad). It governs various aspects of life, including personal behavior, family matters, business transactions, and criminal justice. It serves as a moral and ethical guide for Muslims and aims to promote justice, equality, and the well-being of society as a whole.

Sharia law encompasses a wide range of topics, such as marriage, divorce, inheritance, contracts, and criminal offenses. It places great emphasis on mutual respect, fairness, and compassion. It seeks to protect individual rights and promote

social welfare, encouraging charitable acts, and helping those in need.

Under Sharia law in Iran, women have certain rights and responsibilities, but it's important to note that interpretations and implementations can vary. Here's a general overview:

1. **Life**: Women in Iran have the right to life and personal safety, just like men. However, certain behaviors or choices that are considered against Islamic principles may face stricter punishments or societal pressures.
2. **Education**: Women have access to education in Iran, and there are no legal restrictions on their right to education. However, societal factors and cultural norms can sometimes limit educational opportunities for women, particularly in more conservative areas.

3. **Marriage:** Under Sharia law, women have the right to consent to marriage and cannot be forced into marriage against their will. However, certain legal and cultural practices can undermine this right in some cases. Polygamy is allowed in Iran, but a man must obtain permission from a court and prove his ability to treat all wives equally.
4. **Inheritance**: Sharia law prescribes specific rules for inheritance. In Iran, women generally have the right to inherit property, but the share they receive can be different from that of men. For example, a daughter may receive half the share of a son. However, it's worth noting that recent legal reforms in Iran have aimed to address gender disparities in inheritance rights.

It's important to remember that these are general points, and the actual lived experiences of Iranian women can vary depending on various factors such as regional customs, socio-economic status, and personal circumstances.

Medical Education and Healthcare System Delivery:

The current quota system in the Islamic Republic of Iran aims to promote equal opportunities for underrepresented groups in medical school admission. The quota system intends a certain number of seats for specific categories of applicants, including students from rural areas, ethnic minorities, and individuals with disabilities which in reality is ignored and overlooked. The purpose of this system is to address presumed historical inequalities and increase access to higher education for marginalized populations.

The specific details of the quota system can vary from year to year, but generally, it involves allocating a certain percentage of seats in medical schools to applicants from these underrepresented groups. For example, a certain percentage of seats may be reserved for students from rural areas, regardless of their performance in the entrance exams, merit, and educational aptitude. However, the Islamic Republic ignores its mandated policies and instead, a certain number of seats are reserved for individuals who have demonstrated a commitment to the Islamic faith and have a strong religious background.

Additionally, there may be a quota for the children of war martyrs who are given preferential treatment in the admission process.

These policies aim to promote the values and principles of the Islamic Republic of Iran and ensure that individuals with strong religious beliefs have opportunities to pursue professional education regardless of their eligibility, merit, academic aptitude, and passing scores in entrance exams.

As a rule, the quota system is intended to provide opportunities to individuals who may face additional barriers to accessing quality education or achieving high scores in the highly competitive entrance exams. By reserving a certain number of seats for these groups, the system in a free and democratic society aims to create a more diverse and inclusive medical student body.

However, the implementation and specific details of the quota system have been the subject of debate and criticism in Iran. Some argue that the system may compromise merit-based admission and result in a lower standard of education in medical schools. Critics also express concerns that the system may be susceptible to abuse or manipulation, with applicants falsely claiming eligibility for quota seats.

It is important to note that the quota system is just one aspect of the medical school admission process in many countries. Other criteria, such as performance in specific and national exams and academic achievements, also play a significant role in determining admission. The quota system is meant to supplement these criteria and provide opportunities for underrepresented groups, but it does not solely determine admission outcomes Unfortunately none of the above criteria other than Islamic organization affiliation are observed in the Islamic Republic of Iran.

In Iran, like in many countries, disparities in medical school admission exist and can be attributed to various factors. Some of the main disparities in medical school admission in Iran include:

1. Regional Disparities: There is a significant regional imbalance in medical school admission in Iran. Students from wealthier or more developed regions tend to have better access to quality education and resources, which can give them an advantage in the highly competitive medical school entrance exams. As a result, students from less privileged regions may face additional barriers to gaining admission to medical schools.

2. Socioeconomic Disparities: Socioeconomic factors play a significant role in medical school admission disparities. Students from wealthier backgrounds often have access to better preparatory resources, such as private tutoring or specialized coaching classes, which can enhance their performance in entrance exams. On the other hand, students from lower-income families may face financial constraints and lack the resources necessary to compete on an equal footing.

3. Gender Disparities: Gender disparities can also be observed in medical school admission in Iran. While women make up a significant proportion of medical school applicants, there is a notable gender gap in terms of acceptance rates. This is due to various societal and cultural factors that may discourage or limit women's access to higher education, including medical schools.

4. Educational Disparities: Disparities in the quality of pre-university education can significantly impact medical school admission outcomes. Students from schools with limited resources, outdated curricula, and inadequate teaching staff may face challenges in acquiring the necessary knowledge and skills to perform well in entrance exams. This can disproportionately affect students from marginalized communities.

5. Merit vs. Quota System: The existence of quota systems in medical school

admission can contribute to disparities. To promote equal opportunities for underrepresented groups, including students from rural areas or ethnic minorities, a certain number of seats may be reserved. While this aims to address inequalities, it can also create a perception that some students are admitted based on factors other than merit, leading to concerns about fairness and competition.

Addressing these disparities requires a multi-faceted approach:

1. Equal Access to Quality Education: Improve the quality of pre-university education in underserved regions by investing in infrastructure, resources, and qualified teachers. This will help ensure that students from all regions have an equal opportunity to compete for medical school admission.

2. Targeted Support Programs: Implement targeted support programs, such as scholarship initiatives and mentoring programs, to assist students from disadvantaged backgrounds. These programs can provide financial support, guidance, and resources to help students overcome barriers and compete on an equal footing.

3. Awareness and Outreach: Increase awareness about medical school admission requirements, entrance exams, and available support programs among potential applicants. This can be achieved through targeted outreach campaigns, workshops, and information sessions in schools and communities.

4. Reforming Admission Processes: Continuously review and reform the medical school admission processes to ensure they are fair, transparent, and merit-based. This may involve reducing or eliminating quota systems while still considering the need to address historical inequalities and promote diversity.

5. Gender Equality Promotion: Encourage and support women's participation in higher education, including medical schools, through targeted initiatives, scholarships, and awareness campaigns. Address cultural and societal barriers that discourage women from pursuing medical careers.

6. Collaboration and Research: Foster collaboration between educational institutions, government bodies, and relevant stakeholders to research admission disparities and develop evidence-based strategies for addressing them effectively.

By addressing these disparities in medical school admission, Iran can create a more equitable and inclusive healthcare system, ensuring that talented and deserving individuals from all backgrounds have the opportunity to pursue careers in medicine and contribute to the betterment of society

The current quota system in general and in medical education in particular, not only has negatively impacted medical and higher medical education but also has resulted in lower educational and training quality and standard and quality of care delivery.

The Islamic cultural revolution and the applied Islamic criteria and quotas to the selection process and retaining academic staff and teachers have dramatically and negatively impacted the quality of higher medical education, specialty training, and practice of medicine in the country.

Many academic staff and leaders have been forced to retire or have been expunged.

Many of those medical school graduates also received preferential quota placement and entered specialty training without taking the entrance exam, leaving those with higher scores behind closed doors.

The following are the examples of quota-assigned admission to special training for the academic year 2022-2023:

1-Radiology and Nuclear Medicine > 50%2- Orthopedic Surgery > 69% 3-

Cardiovascular Disease > 62%

This trend applies to all training in the country. Rebuilding and remedial needs:

This process is multifaceted and requires large and qualified personnel and a task force. In all three sections, medical school, specialty and residency, and practicing physicians and healthcare.

1. Program Assessment and Identification:

- Conduct a thorough assessment of the current situation, including the admission process, curriculum, and competency levels of the affected physicians.

- Identify the specific religious or political connections that influenced their admission and evaluate the impact on their medical knowledge and skills.

- Collaborate with local healthcare authorities, educational institutions, and professional associations to develop a targeted retraining program.

2. Preparatory Courses:

- Offer preparatory courses to bridge knowledge gaps in basic medical sciences, such as anatomy, physiology, biochemistry, and pharmacology.

- Provide comprehensive lectures, interactive sessions, and practical demonstrations to ensure a strong foundation in essential medical concepts.

- Utilize modern teaching methodologies, including case-based learning and problem-solving exercises, to promote critical thinking and clinicalreasoning.

3. Clinical Training and Skill Development:

- Arrange clinical rotations and internships in reputable healthcare institutions to provide hands-on experience under the guidance of experienced physicians.

- Focus on enhancing clinical skills, including history taking, physical examination, diagnostic reasoning, and evidence-based treatment planning.

- Provide opportunities for physicians to observe and participate in various medical procedures, surgeries, and specialized clinics relevant to their chosen specialties.

4. Specialty-Specific Education:

- Tailor the retraining program to each physician's desired specialty, such as internal medicine, surgery, pediatrics, obstetrics, and gynecology.

- Offer specialty-specific lectures, workshops, and case discussions to deepen their understanding and practical skills in their chosen field.

- Engage specialists from various disciplines to provide comprehensive and up-to-date knowledge, fostering a multidisciplinary approach.

5. Professional Ethics and Communication Skills:

- Conduct workshops and seminars on medical ethics, professionalism, and effective communication skills.

- Emphasize the importance of patient-centered care, cultural sensitivity, and respect for diverse religious and political beliefs.

- Engage physicians in role-playing exercises, simulated patient interactions, and discussions on challenging ethical dilemmas to enhance their decision-making skills.

6. Continuous Medical Education:

- Establish a framework for continuous medical education to ensure physicians stay updated with the latest medical advancements and evidence-based practices.

- Provide access to online resources, medical journals, conferences, and workshops to support ongoing learning and professional growth.

- Encourage physicians to participate in research activities, present scientific papers, and contribute to medical literature to foster intellectual development.

7. Mentorship and Support:

- Assign experienced physicians as mentors to provide guidance, support, and career advice throughout the retraining program.

- Facilitate regular mentorship sessions to discuss challenges, set goals, and monitor progress, ensuring personalized support for each physician.

- Foster a supportive community by organizing networking events, peer-to-peer learning opportunities, and mentor-led discussions.

8. Program Evaluation and Monitoring:

- Establish an evaluation framework to assess the effectiveness of the retraining program and monitor the progress of participating physicians.

- Collect feedback from participants, mentors, and healthcare employers to identify strengths, weaknesses, and areas requiring improvement.

- Utilize evaluation results to refine the program, update curriculum content, adjust teaching methodologies, and address emerging needs.

9. Collaboration and Partnerships:

- Collaborate with local and international stakeholders, including healthcare institutions, professional associations, NGOs, and funding agencies.

- Seek partnerships with reputable medical schools or organizations to enhance program credibility and provide additional resources.

- Engage with policymakers and advocacy groups to address systemic issues and promote merit-based admission processes in medical education.

10. Sustainability and Long-Term Impact:

- Foster local ownership by involving local healthcare authorities, medical institutions, and professional associations in program planning and implementation.

- Develop a sustainability plan to ensure the program's continuity beyond the initial retraining phase, including strategies for financial support and resource management.

- Monitor the long-term impact of the program by tracking the professional success, career progression, and contributions of the retrained physicians to the healthcare sector.

By implementing this comprehensive retraining program, we aim to empower physicians who were admitted based on religious or political connections to acquire the necessary medical knowledge, skills, and ethical values. This program seeks to bridge the educational gaps and ensure that these physicians can provide high-quality, evidence-based healthcare, thereby improving the overall healthcare system in third-world countries.

Allied Health Professional Remedial and Retraining:

This is a comprehensive program to retrain allied healthcare professionals in Iran transition and freedom who were admitted to professional schools based on religious or political rather than merit or aptitude:

1. Program Assessment and Planning:

- Conduct a thorough assessment of the current situation, including the admission process, curriculum, and competency levels of the allied healthcare professionals.

- Identify the specific religious or political connections that affected their admission and evaluate the impact on their knowledge and skills.

- Collaborate with local healthcare authorities, educational institutions, and professional associations to develop a comprehensive retraining program.

2. Remedial Education and Skill Development:

- Offer foundational courses to bridge knowledge gaps in basic healthcare sciences, including anatomy, physiology, pharmacology, and medical terminology.

- Provide specialized training to enhance practical skills and competence in their respective allied healthcare fields, such as nursing, medical technology, or physiotherapy.

- Utilize a combination of classroom lectures, hands-on training, simulation exercises, and practical applications to reinforce learning.

3. Professional Ethics and Values:

- Conduct workshops and discussions on professional ethics, emphasizing the importance of merit-based admission, equality, and patient-centered care.

- Facilitate sessions on cultural sensitivity, diversity, and respect for religious or political beliefs while ensuring unbiased and evidence-based healthcare practice.

- Encourage open dialogue and critical thinking to challenge preconceived notions and promote ethical decision-making in healthcare settings.

4. Clinical Experience and Practical Exposure:

- Arrange clinical rotations, internships, or apprenticeships in reputable healthcare facilities to provide hands-on experience under the guidance of experienced professionals.

- Encourage active participation in patient care, diagnostic procedures, treatment planning, and interprofessional collaboration to develop practical skills and confidence.

- Monitor and evaluate performance during clinical experiences to provide constructive feedback and identify areas for improvement.

5. Leadership and Management Skills:

- Offer training in leadership and management skills to equip allied healthcare professionals with the ability to lead teams, ensure quality care, and advocate for patient rights.

- Develop courses on healthcare administration, resource management, and effective communication to enhance their roles as future leaders in the healthcare sector.

- Provide opportunities for project management and quality improvement initiatives to foster innovation and enhance the ability to address healthcare challenges.

6. Continuous Professional Development:

- Establish a framework for ongoing professional development to ensure the retraining professionals stay updated with advancements in their fields.

- Provide access to relevant continuing education resources, online courses, conferences, and workshops to support lifelong learning.

- Encourage participation in research activities, publication opportunities, and knowledge-sharing platforms to foster professional growth and contribute to the healthcare community.

7. Mentorship and Support:

- Assign experienced allied healthcare professionals as mentors to provide guidance, support, and career advice throughout the retraining program.

- Facilitate regular mentorship sessions to discuss challenges, set goals, and monitor progress, ensuring personalized support for each retraining professional.

- Foster a supportive community by organizing networking events, peer-to-peer learning opportunities, and mentor-led discussions.

8. Program Evaluation and Monitoring:

- Establish an evaluation framework to monitor the effectiveness of the retraining program and assess the retraining professional progress.

- Collect feedback from participants, mentors, and healthcare employers to identify strengths, weaknesses, and areas requiring improvement.

- Use evaluation results to refine the program, update curriculum content, adjust teaching methodologies, and address emerging needs.

9. Collaboration and Partnerships:

- Collaborate with local and international stakeholders, including healthcare institutions, professional associations, NGOs, and funding agencies.

- Seek partnerships with reputable educational institutions or organizations to enhance program credibility and provide additional resources.

- Engage with policymakers and advocacy groups to address systemic issues and promote merit-based admission processes in allied healthcare education.

10. Sustainability and Long-Term Impact:

- Foster local ownership by involving local healthcare authorities, educational institutions, and professional associations in program planning and implementation.

- Develop a sustainability plan to ensure the program's continuity beyond the initial retraining phase, including strategies for financial support and resource management.

- Monitor the long-term impact of the program by tracking the professional success, career progression, and contributions of the retraining professionals to the healthcare sector.

Implementing this comprehensive retraining program requires strong collaboration among various stakeholders, meticulous planning, and ongoing evaluation. By addressing the educational gaps caused by religious or political connections, this program aims to empower allied healthcare professionals to deliver high-quality, patient-centered care based on merit and aptitude.

Pharmacy and related Industries:

Here is a comprehensive program to retrain pharmacists in Iran during the transition and after people victory who were admitted to professional schools based on religious or political connections rather than merit or aptitude:

1. Program Orientation and Needs Assessment:

- Conduct an orientation session to explain the program's objectives, expectations, and benefits to the pharmacists.

- Administer a comprehensive needs assessment to identify their strengths, weaknesses, and areas requiring improvement.

- Gather data on their pharmacy education background, pharmaceutical knowledge, clinical skills, and personal goals.

2. Core Pharmaceutical Knowledge Enhancement:

- Provide intensive training in core pharmaceutical knowledge, including pharmacology, pharmaceutics, pharmacokinetics, and pharmacotherapy, to ensure a strong foundation.

- Offer specialized courses and workshops to update pharmacists on the latest drug information, evidence-based practice, and global health issues.

- Utilize interactive teaching methods, case studies, and practical exercises to enhance critical thinking and problem-solving skills.

3. Clinical Skills Development:

- Conduct hands-on training sessions to improve clinical skills, including medication dispensing, drug interaction screening, patient counseling, and medication therapy management.

- Provide simulated patient encounters and pharmacy simulations to practice and refine clinical skills in a controlled environment.

- Offer guidance on effective communication with patients, healthcare providers, and other members of the healthcare team to ensure patient-centered care.

4. Pharmaceutical Care and Patient Safety:

- Emphasize the importance of pharmaceutical care and patient safety in the practice of pharmacy.

- Provide training on medication reconciliation, adverse drug event reporting, medication error prevention, and quality assurance in pharmacy practice.

- Encourage pharmacists to develop patient monitoring plans, assess therapeutic outcomes, and collaborate with healthcare teams to optimize patient care.

5. Specialized Training and Continuing Education:

- Develop specialized training modules based on the pharmacists' areas of interest or the healthcare needs of their communities.

- Offer continuing pharmacy education (CPE) courses, conferences, and workshops to keep the pharmacists updated with the latest research, guidelines, and best practices.

- Collaborate with local and international pharmacy experts to deliver specialized training and share their expertise.

6. Ethical and Professional Development:

- Conduct sessions on pharmacy ethics, professional integrity, and patient confidentiality to reinforce the importance of ethical conduct in pharmacy practice.

- Promote evidence-based practice and encourage pharmacists to base their clinical decisions on scientific research and patient well-being.

- Facilitate discussions on the impact of religious or political influences on the pharmaceutical sector and emphasize the need for unbiased and patient-centered care.

7. Mentoring and Individual Support:

- Assign experienced pharmacists as mentors to provide one-on-one guidance, support, and career advice to the retraining pharmacists.

- Conduct regular mentorship sessions to address individual concerns, monitor progress, and provide feedback on clinical skills and professional development.

- Encourage retraining pharmacists to seek advice and share experiences with their mentors, promoting a supportive learning environment.

8. Practical Exposure and Internships:

- Collaborate with local healthcare institutions, community pharmacies, and pharmaceutical companies to provide practical exposure and internships.

- Offer opportunities to work alongside experienced pharmacists, observe pharmaceutical processes, and participate in patient care under supervision.

- Arrange internships in various settings, such as hospitals, retail pharmacies, pharmaceutical manufacturing, and regulatory bodies, to provide well-rounded experiential learning.

9. Continuous Assessment and Progress Monitoring:

- Implement regular assessments, exams, and evaluations to track the progress of retraining pharmacists and identify areas needing improvement.

- Provide constructive feedback to help them understand their strengths and weaknesses, enabling them to work on their clinical skills and professional growth.

- Use data and feedback to adapt the program and address the evolving needs of the retraining pharmacists.

10. Networking and Collaboration:

- Establish a network of retraining pharmacists to foster collaboration, knowledge sharing, and peer support.

- Organize pharmacy conferences, webinars, and seminars to facilitate networking opportunities with healthcare professionals from various specialties and countries.

- Encourage retraining pharmacists to engage in research projects, publications, and quality improvement initiatives to contribute to the pharmacy community.

11. Program Evaluation and Improvement:

- Regularly evaluate the program's effectiveness through feedback from retraining pharmacists, mentors, and healthcare professionals.

- Analyze data and make necessary adjustments to the curriculum, teaching methodologies, and program structure to address emergingneeds.

- Collaborate with local governments, healthcare organizations, and international partners to secure funding, resources, and support for program sustainability and expansion.

Implementing this comprehensive program would require collaboration with relevant stakeholders, including pharmacy schools, healthcare institutions, professional associations, and funding agencies. It is essential to ensure the availability of adequate resources, qualified trainers, and ongoing support to maximize the impact and success of the pharmacist retraining program.

Nursing and Support Staff:

This is a comprehensive program to retrain nurses and support staff after the uprising and victory in Iran who like many other professionals were admitted to professional schools based on religious or political connections rather than merit or aptitude:

1. Program Orientation and Needs Assessment:

- Conduct an orientation session to explain the program's objectives, expectations, and benefits to the nurses.

- Administer a comprehensive needs assessment to identify their strengths, weaknesses, and areas requiring improvement.

- Gather data on their nursing education background, clinical skills, and personal goals.

2. Core Nursing Knowledge Enhancement:

- Provide intensive training in core nursing knowledge, including anatomy, physiology, pharmacology, and nursing theories, to ensure a strong foundation.

- Offer specialized courses and workshops to update nurses on the latest nursing practices, evidence-based care, and global health issues.

- Utilize interactive teaching methods, case studies, and practical exercises to enhance critical thinking and clinical reasoning skills.

3. Clinical Skills Development:

- Conduct hands-on training sessions to improve clinical skills, including patient assessment, medication administration, wound care, and infection control.

- Provide simulated patient encounters and nursing simulations to practice and refine clinical skills in a controlled environment.

- Offer guidance on effective communication with patients, families, and healthcare teams, empathy, and cultural sensitivity to foster patient-centered care.

4. Specialized Training and Continuing Education:

- Develop specialized training modules based on the nurses' areas of interest or the healthcare needs of their communities.

- Offer continuing nursing education (CNE) courses, conferences, and workshops to keep the nurses updated with the latest nursing research, guidelines, and best practices.

- Collaborate with local and international nursing experts to deliver specialized training and share their expertise.

5. Ethical and Professional Development:

- Conduct sessions on nursing ethics, professional integrity, and patient advocacy to reinforce the importance of ethical conduct in nursing.

- Promote evidence-based nursing practice and encourage nurses to base their clinical decisions on scientific research and patient well-being.

- Facilitate discussions on the impact of religious or political influences on healthcare and emphasize the need for unbiased nursing care.

6. Mentoring and Individual Support:

- Assign experienced nurses as mentors to provide one-on-one guidance, support, and career advice to the retraining nurses.

- Conduct regular mentorship sessions to address individual concerns, monitor progress, and provide feedback on clinical skills and professional development.

- Encourage retraining nurses to seek advice and share experiences with their mentors, promoting a supportive learning environment.

7. Practical Exposure and Clinical Rotations:

- Collaborate with local healthcare institutions to provide practical exposure and clinical rotations in different healthcare settings.

- Offer opportunities to work alongside experienced nurses, observe procedures, and participate in patient care under supervision.

- Arrange rotations in various healthcare settings, such as hospitals, clinics, community health centers, and home care, to provide a well-rounded clinical experience.

8. Continuous Assessment and Progress Monitoring:

- Implement regular assessments, exams, and clinical evaluations to track the progress of retraining nurses and identify areas needing improvement.

- Provide constructive feedback to help them understand their strengths and weaknesses, enabling them to work on their clinical skills and professional growth.

- Use data and feedback to adapt the program and address the evolving needs of the retraining nurses.

9. Networking and Collaboration:

- Establish a network of retraining nurses to foster collaboration, knowledge sharing, and peer support.

- Organize nursing conferences, webinars, and seminars to facilitate networking opportunities with healthcare professionals from various specialties and countries.

- Encourage retraining nurses to engage in research projects, publications, and quality improvement initiatives to contribute to the nursing community.

10. Program Evaluation and Improvement:

- Regularly evaluate the program's effectiveness through feedback from retraining nurses, mentors, and healthcare professionals.

- Analyze data and make necessary adjustments to the curriculum, teaching methodologies, and program structure to address emerging needs.

- Collaborate with local governments, healthcare organizations, and international partners to secure funding, resources, and support for program sustainability and expansion.

-

Implementing this comprehensive program would require collaboration with relevant stakeholders, including nursing schools, healthcare institutions, professional associations, and funding agencies. It is essential to ensure the availability of adequate resources, qualified trainers, and ongoing support to maximize the impact and success of the nurse retraining program.

Practicing Physicians in different settings; Academic, private government/charity sectors:

1. Program Orientation and Needs Assessment:

- Conduct an orientation session to explain the program's objectives, expectations, and benefits to the physicians.

- Administer a comprehensive needs assessment to identify their strengths, weaknesses, and areas requiring improvement.

- Gather data on their medical education background, clinical skills, and personal goals.

2. Core Medical Knowledge Enhancement:

- Provide intensive training in core medical knowledge, including anatomy, physiology, pharmacology, and pathology, to ensure a strong foundation.

- Offer specialized courses and workshops to update physicians on the latest medical advancements, evidence-based practices, and global health issues.

- Utilize interactive teaching methods, case studies, and practical exercises to enhance critical thinking and clinical reasoning skills.

3. Clinical Skills Development:

- Conduct hands-on training sessions to improve clinical skills, including history taking, physical examination, diagnosis, and treatment planning.

- Provide simulated patient encounters and medical simulations to practice and refine clinical skills in a controlled environment.

- Offer guidance on effective communication with patients, empathy, and cultural sensitivity to foster patient-centered care.

4. Specialized Training and Continuing Medical Education:

- Develop specialized training modules based on the physicians of interest or the healthcare needs of their communities.

- Offer continuing medical education (CME) courses, conferences, and workshops to keep the physicians updated with the latest medical research, guidelines, and best practices.

- Collaborate with local and international medical experts to deliver specialized training and sharing their expertise.

5. Ethical and Professional Development:

- Conduct sessions on medical ethics, professional integrity, and patient confidentiality to reinforce the importance of ethical conduct in healthcare.

- Promote evidence-based medicine and encourage physicians to base their clinical decisions on scientific research and patient well-being.

- Facilitate discussions on the impact of religious or political influences on healthcare and emphasize the need for unbiased medical practice.

6. Mentoring and Individual Support:

- Assign experienced physicians as mentors to provide one-on-one guidance, support, and career advice to the retraining physicians.

- Conduct regular mentorship sessions to address individual concerns, monitor progress, and provide feedback on clinical skills and professional development.

- Encourage retraining physicians to seek advice and share experiences with their mentors, promoting a supportive learning environment.

7. Practical Exposure and Clinical Rotations:

- Collaborate with local healthcare institutions to provide practical exposure and clinical rotations in different medical specialties.

- Offer opportunities to work alongside experienced physicians, observe procedures, and participate in patient care under supervision.

- Arrange rotations in various healthcare settings, including hospitals, primary care clinics, and community health centers, to provide a well-rounded clinical experience.

8. Continuous Assessment and Progress Monitoring:

- Implement regular assessments, exams, and clinical evaluations to track the progress of retraining physicians and identify areas needing improvement.

- Provide constructive feedback to help them understand their strengths and weaknesses, enabling them to work on their clinical skills and professional growth.

- Use data and feedback to adapt the program and address the evolving needs of the retraining physicians.

- Networking and Collaboration:
  Establish a network of retraining physicians to collaborate,

knowledge sharing, and peer support.

- Organize medical conferences, webinars, and seminars to facilitate networking opportunities with healthcare professionals from various specialties and countries.

- Encourage retraining physicians to engage in research projects, publications, and quality improvement initiatives to contribute to the medical community.

9. Program Evaluation and Improvement:

- Regularly evaluate the program's effectiveness through feedback from retraining physicians, mentors, and healthcare professionals.

- Analyze data and make necessary adjustments to the curriculum, teaching methodologies, and program structure to address emergingneeds.

- Collaborate with local governments, healthcare organizations, and international partners to secure funding, resources, and support for program sustainability and expansion.

Implementing this comprehensive program would require collaboration with relevant stakeholders, including medical institutions, professional associations, and funding agencies. It is crucial to ensure the availability of adequate resources, qualified trainers, and ongoing support to maximize the impact and success of the physician retraining program.

Carrier Practicing Healthcare In Different Settings And Specialties:

1. Program Orientation and Needs Assessment:

- Conduct an orientation session to explain the program's objectives, expectations, and benefits to the graduates.

- Administer a comprehensive needs assessment to identify their strengths, weaknesses, and areas requiring improvement.

- Gather data on their educational background, professional aspirations, and personal goals.

2. Remedial Education and Foundation Building:

- Provide remedial classes in fundamental subjects (e.g., mathematics, science, language skills) to fill knowledge gaps and ensure a strong foundation.

- Offer specialized courses to enhance critical thinking, problem-solving, and analytical skills necessary for their respective professions.

- Incorporate interactive teaching methods, practical exercises, and group discussions to engage and motivate the graduates.

3. Skill Enhancement and Professional Training:

- Develop a curriculum that focuses on the specific professional skills required in their field of study.

- Offer specialized courses and workshops to strengthen technical knowledge and practical competencies.

- Provide hands-on training, simulations, and real-life case studies to bridge the gap between theory and application.

- Collaborate with industry experts and professionals to deliver guest lectures, share practical insights, and offer guidance.

4. Ethical and Professional Development:

- Conduct sessions on professional ethics, integrity, and responsibility, emphasizing the importance of merit-based practices.

- Foster a culture of integrity, accountability, and transparency by promoting ethical decision-making and professional conduct.

- Organize workshops on effective communication, teamwork, and leadership skills to enhance their professional capabilities.

5. Mentoring and Individual Support:

- Assign mentors who are experienced professionals in their respective fields to provide personalized guidance and support.

- Conduct regular mentorship sessions to address individual concerns, monitor progress, and provide career guidance.

- Encourage graduates to seek advice and share experiences with their mentors, promoting a supportive learning environment.

6. Practical Exposure and Internships:

- Collaborate with local organizations, companies, and government bodies to provide practical exposure and internship opportunities.

- Facilitate internships, apprenticeships, or on-the-job training to enhance their practical skills and gain real-world experience.

- Encourage graduates to actively participate in community service initiatives, fostering a sense of social responsibility.

7. Continuous Assessment and Progress Monitoring:

- Implement regular assessments, exams, and performance evaluations to track their progress and identify areas needing improvement.

- Provide constructive feedback to help graduates understand their strengths and weaknesses, enabling them to work on their professional development.

- Use data and feedback to adapt the program and address the evolving needs of the graduates.

8. Networking and Alumni Engagement:

- Establish an alumni network to connect graduates with professionals, mentors, and peers in their field.

- Organize networking events, conferences, and seminars to facilitate knowledge sharing and professional connections.

- Encourage alumni to contribute back to the program by mentoring new participants or providing guest lectures.

9. Continuous Learning and Growth:

- Emphasize the importance of lifelong learning and professional development to ensure graduates stay updated with industry trends.

- Provide resources, access to online courses, and learning materials to support their ongoing growth and skill enhancement.

- Encourage graduates to pursue higher education, research opportunities, or certifications to further advance in their careers.

10. Program Evaluation and Improvement:

- Regularly evaluate the program's effectiveness through feedback from graduates, mentors, and industry professionals.

- Analyze data and make necessary adjustments to the curriculum, teaching methodologies, and program structure.

- Collaborate with stakeholders to secure funding, resources, and support for the program sustainability and expansion.

Remember, this comprehensive program outline serves as a starting point, and the actual implementation would require thorough planning, collaboration with relevant organizations, and securing necessary resources.

Healthcare Emergencies:
Arm Forces' role

The role of army and military forces in healthcare crisis management in both urban and rural areas can be significant. Here are some key roles they can play:

1. Emergency response and disaster management: The army and military forces have the training, resources, and logistical capabilities to respond quickly to healthcare crises, such as natural disasters, pandemics, or other emergencies. They can provide immediate assistance in setting up field hospitals, triage centers, and temporary medical facilities in both urban and rural areas.

2. Infrastructure support: The army can assist in rebuilding or repairing damaged healthcare infrastructure, such as hospitals, clinics, and medical facilities, in post-crisis situations. They can provide manpower, equipment, and expertise to expedite the restoration of healthcare services.

3. Transportation and logistics: Military forces have well-established transportation and logistics capabilities. They can assist in the transportation of medical personnel, equipment, supplies, and patients, especially in remote or hard-to-reach rural areas. This is particularly crucial during healthcare crises when the regular transportation system may be disrupted.

4. Security and protection: During healthcare crises, maintaining law and order is essential to ensure the safety of healthcare professionals, patients, and medical facilities. The army and military forces can provide security and protection to healthcare workers, medical facilities, and supply routes, particularly in conflict-affected areas.

5. Humanitarian aid and outreach: Military forces often have access to resources and capabilities to provide humanitarian aid and outreach in healthcare crises. They can distribute essential supplies, provide medical assistance, and support vaccination campaigns in both urban and rural areas, especially when there are limited healthcare resources available.

6. Training and capacity building: The army and military forces can contribute to training healthcare personnel in disaster response, emergency medical care, and crisis management. They can share their expertise and experiences with healthcare professionals, community health workers, and volunteers to enhance their readiness and capabilities during future healthcare crises.

7. Coordination and collaboration: The army can play a crucial role in coordinating and collaborating with other stakeholders, including government agencies, non-governmental organizations (NGOs), and international partners. They can establish joint command centers, facilitate information sharing, and ensure effective coordination among various actors involved in healthcare crisis management.

However, it is important to note that the involvement of the army and military forces in healthcare crisis management should be governed by clear guidelines and principles. They should work in close collaboration with healthcare authorities and abide by medical ethics to ensure that healthcare interventions are provided in a manner that prioritizes the well-being and dignity of affected populations.

Integration of Advanced Technology in Post-Revolution Iran Healthcare System and Medical Education

Five Years of strategic planning

In recent years, the rapid advancement of technology has brought about significant changes in various industries, including medicine. Applicable technology, specifically in the field of medicine, refers to the innovative tools, devices, and software that are being developed and applied to improve healthcare outcomes, enhance patient care, and streamline medical processes. From artificial intelligence and machine learning to telemedicine and wearable devices, these technologies have the potential to revolutionize the way healthcare is delivered and experienced. In this article, we will explore some of the most promising and impactful technologies that are transforming the medical landscape and delve into their applications and benefits.

The future of medicine and technology is incredibly exciting and holds great potential for improving healthcare outcomes. Here are a few areas where we can expect significant advancements:

1. Personalized Medicine: With advancements in genomics and molecular biology, medicine is increasingly becoming tailored to individuals. Genetic testing and analysis can provide insights into an individual's susceptibility to certain diseases, allowing for targeted prevention and treatment strategies.
2. Telemedicine and Remote Patient Monitoring: Technology enables doctors to remotely monitor patients and provide consultations, especially for those who live in remote areas or have limited mobility. This can greatly improve access to healthcare and reduce the burden of in-person visits.
3. Artificial Intelligence (AI) in Healthcare: AI has the potential to revolutionize medicine by analyzing vast amounts of data, identifying patterns, and assisting in diagnosis and treatment decisions. Machine learning algorithms can help predict disease progression, optimize treatment plans, and even automate certain medical procedures.
4. Robotics and Automation: Robotic technologies are being developed to assist in surgeries, allowing for more precise and minimally invasive procedures. Additionally, robotics can aid in physical therapy and rehabilitation, enabling faster recovery for patients.
5. Wearable Devices and Sensors: The rise of wearable technology, such as smartwatches and fitness trackers, has already begun to impact healthcare. These devices can monitor vital signs, track activity levels, and provide real-time health feedback, empowering individuals to take proactive steps toward better health.

6. These are just a few glimpses into the future of medicine and technology. The possibilities are vast, and ongoing advancements will continue to transform the healthcare landscape, improving patient care and outcomes.

IBM Watson is a powerful example of how technology, specifically artificial intelligence (AI), is being harnessed to revolutionize medicine. Developed by IBM, Watson is an AI platform that utilizes machine learning and natural language processing capabilities to process and interpret vast amounts of data.

In the field of medicine, Watson has shown immense potential in several areas:

1. Clinical Decision Support: Watson can analyze patient data, including medical records, lab results, and research papers, to provide evidence-based recommendations to healthcare providers. This assists in diagnosing complex conditions, suggesting treatment options, and avoiding potential errors or oversights.
2. Oncology: Watson for Oncology is a specialized application of Watson that helps oncologists in cancer care. By analyzing vast amounts of medical literature, clinical guidelines, and patient data, Watson can provide personalized treatment options based on a patient's unique genetic and clinical profile. This can help doctors make more informed decisions and provide targeted therapies.
3. Drug Discovery and Development: Watson's capabilities extend to pharmaceutical research and development. By analyzing large amounts of scientific literature, clinical trials, and genetic data, Watson can identify potential drug targets, predict drug interactions, and accelerate the drug discovery process. This has the potential to significantly reduce the time and cost involved in bringing new drugs to market.
4. Medical Education and Training: Watson's AI capabilities are also being utilized in medical education. By providing access to a vast knowledge base and utilizing interactive learning tools, Watson can help medical students and professionals stay updated with the latest research and guidelines. It can also assist in simulating clinical scenarios and offering virtual patient consultations, aiding in training and skill development.
5. IBM Watson's integration into healthcare is an ongoing process, and its potential continues to expand. While there are still challenges to address, such as data privacy and integration with existing healthcare systems, Watson stands as a remarkable example of how AI can augment healthcare professionals' expertise, enhance patient care, and contribute to medical advancements.

Role of Technology in Medical Education

Technology plays a crucial role in transforming medical education by enhancing learning experiences, promoting collaboration, and keeping up with advancements in healthcare. Here are some key roles that technology plays in medical education:

1. Access to information: Technology provides instant access to a vast amount of medical information, research papers, textbooks, and online resources. Medical students can use online databases, e-books, and medical apps to access the latest information, study materials, and clinical guidelines, enabling them to stay updated on medical knowledge.

2. Simulation and virtual learning: Technology enables the use of virtual reality (VR) and augmented reality (AR) to create realistic medical simulations. Medical students can practice procedures, surgeries, and patient interactions in a safe and controlled environment, enhancing their skills and confidence before real-life patient encounters.

3. E-learning platforms: Learning management systems (LMS) and online platforms facilitate interactive and self-paced learning. Medical students can access lectures, videos, quizzes, and discussion forums, providing flexibility in their learning journey. These platforms also enable educators to track student progress and provide personalized feedback.

4. Collaborative learning: Technology fosters collaboration among medical students, educators, and healthcare professionals. Online platforms, video conferencing, and discussion forums facilitate virtual teamwork, case-based learning, and peer-to-peer collaboration. This enhances critical thinking, problem-solving, and communication skills among future healthcare professionals.

5. Remote learning and telemedicine: Technology enables remote learning, allowing medical students to access lectures, workshops, and conferences from anywhere. Telemedicine platforms also provide opportunities for students to observe virtual patient consultations and participate in remote clinical rotations, expanding their exposure to different medical specialties and patient populations.

6. Digital anatomy and visualization tools: Technology offers 3D modeling, digital anatomy atlases, and interactive visualization tools that enhance the understanding of complex anatomical structures and physiological processes. These tools provide a more immersive and interactive learning experience compared to traditional textbooks and diagrams.

7. Mobile apps and point-of-care tools: Medical apps and point-of-care tools assist medical students in quick reference, decision-making, and clinical reasoning. From drug reference guides to medical calculators and clinical guidelines, these apps provide readily accessible information to support learning and patient care.

8. Data analysis and research: Technology enables medical students to analyze large datasets, perform research, and contribute to evidence-based medicine. Access to electronic health records (EHRs) and research databases allows students to develop research skills, conduct statistical analyses, and contribute to medical advancements.

Incorporating technology in medical education enhances engagement, improves clinical skills, promotes lifelong learning, and prepares future healthcare professionals for the evolving healthcare landscape. However, it is essential to balance the integration of technology with hands-on clinical experiences and ethical considerations to ensure comprehensive and patient-centered education.

Five-Year Strategic Planning

Year 1: Assessment and Planning

- Conduct a comprehensive assessment of the current healthcare system, identifying areas where technology integration can make the most impact.

- Engage with healthcare professionals, administrators, and IT experts to gather insights and understand their needs and challenges.

- Develop a strategic plan that outlines the goals, objectives, and timeline for integrating technology into the healthcare system.

- Allocate resources and establish a dedicated team to oversee the implementation process.

Year 2: Infrastructure Development

- Upgrade the existing IT infrastructure to support the integration of technology.

- Invest in robust data storage and security systems to ensure patient information is protected.

- Implement electronic health record (EHR) systems across all healthcare facilities to streamline data management and improve accessibility for healthcare providers.

- Establish secure and reliable networks to facilitate seamless communication and data sharing between different healthcare entities.

Year 3: Adoption of Telemedicine

- Implement telemedicine platforms and technologies to enable remote consultations and virtual care.

- Train healthcare professionals on how to effectively use telemedicine tools and provide remote care to patients.

- Collaborate with insurance providers to develop reimbursement policies for telemedicine services.

- Expand telemedicine services to reach underserved areas and improve access to healthcare.

Year 4: Integration of Artificial Intelligence (AI)

- Explore and implement AI algorithms to assist in diagnostics, treatment planning, and data analysis.

- Develop partnerships with AI technology providers to integrate their solutions into the healthcare system.

- Train healthcare professionals on how to effectively use AI-powered tools and leverage them for improved patient outcomes.

- Continuously monitor and evaluate the impact of AI integration on healthcare processes and patient care.

Year 5: Adoption of Wearable Devices and Remote Monitoring

- Implement wearable devices that can collect and transmit patient data in real-time, such as heart rate, blood pressure, and glucose levels.

- Integrate remote monitoring technologies to enable continuous monitoring of patients with chronic conditions.

- Establish protocols and guidelines for healthcare providers to interpret and respond to data collected from wearable devices.

- Collaborate with pharmaceutical companies to leverage wearable technology for medication adherence and clinical trials.

Throughout the five-year strategic planning, it is crucial to prioritize cybersecurity measures, regularly update technology systems, and continuously assess the impact of integrated technology on healthcare outcomes. Additionally, fostering a culture of innovation, training and supporting healthcare professionals in adopting and effectively utilizing technology, and ensuring patient privacy and consent are essential considerations.

General Health and Healthcare

Overview

Health systems as defined as healthcare systems have local and regional specifications and are determined by each country's governing and political structure.

There is, however, an international consensus in definition, component, and infrastructure adopted and modified by each respective country and community based on population, cultural, religious, and political structures.

In general, the health systems are ideated as health policy and management or healthcare systems and management.

In international use and consensus, the health systems policy and management encompass a common field of healthcare systems, public health systems, administration, healthcare administrators, hospitals and hospital networks, medical education and research, leadership, and social determinants.

The above fields are further defined by applicable subsets, divisions and subdivisions, sections, and nations.

In general, the cost and expenditure of health systems and the sustainability of health systems are allocated through national health budgets derived from the national Gross Domestic Product (GPD).

Rationing and Access to Healthcare:

One of the most important of the healthcare system is the delivery and accessibility of the healthcare systems.

Healthcare delivery like many aspects of healthcare systems is addressed and funded by market force and comprehensive build and infrastructures.

Accessibility and rationing of health systems have complex and diversified dimensions which in turn impact how and when people access the healthcare systems and services in different fields of health systems and management.

Delivery and accessibility further way in healthcare systems and policy, when people find that the services they expect and need are not provided, available, or covered by by healthcare systems and public policies.

In many countries and communities, urban and particularly in rural and remote areas with rough terrains and precipitous heights such as Iran, both delivery and accessibility could be problems, difficult, and sometimes near impossible regardless of viable and existing programs.

Another hardship and obstacle to health systems availability and affordability is poorly funded and poorly managed health systems, which impacts the utilization of the services regardless of the financial status and resources of individuals.

Because all health systems services are needed by many at different stages of life and over extended periods and at times urgencies and disastrous circumstances, they can impoverish large sectors of the population but not the most affluent segment of the population.

Another field in healthcare systems is preventive healthcare systems. Utilizing the level and intensity of preventive care provided to the population and preventive measures taken by individuals could strongly predict and determine the health of a community and population.

Medical education and medical and health systems research are also an important field in healthcare systems and management systems. Medical education is a large component of healthcare systems expenditure and long-term investment which directly impacts measures, outcomes, and health systems improvement and dynamics.

Any discussion and reviewing of healthcare systems is not complete without addressing the "access and ratio" in the healthcare system regardless of the related fields.

Although the universal Healthcare systems with different structures are desirable internationally, however, the providing country has to deal with rationing issues.

There are different formats and levels of importance based on the population base and the community's needs.

The more elaborate the universal healthcare system the more government subsidies and rationing issues and negative effects on services.

Current Islamic Republic of Iran Health Systems:

It is of utmost importance to discuss and perceive this section with an air of cautiousness and grain of assault. Like many of IR's other claims, domestically and internationally, the introduction of the healthcare system is misleading and farce.

Islamic Republic constitution:

Article 3

To attain the objectives specified in Article 2, the government of the Islamic Republic of Iran has the duty of directing all its resources to the following goals:

1. the creation of a favorable environment for the growth of moral virtues based on faith and piety and the struggle against all forms of vice and corruption;
2. raising the level of public awareness in all areas, through the proper use of the press, mass media, and other means;
3. free education and physical training for everyone at all levels, and the facilitation and

expansion of higher education;

4. strengthening the spirit of inquiry, investigation, and innovation in all areas of science, technology, and culture, as well as Islamic studies, by establishing research centers and encouraging researchers;

There are very limited articles in the constitution that directly address the healthcare system requirements and mandates rather than emphasizing on Islamic health and hygiene in a very vague terminology. The following are the articles that might or might not address healthcare

"Through the creation of Islamic social infrastructures, all the elements of humanity that hitherto served the multifaceted foreign exploitation shall regain their true identity and human rights. As a part of this process, it is only natural that women should benefit from a particularly large augmentation of their rights, because of the greater oppression that they suffered under the Taghuti regime."

"The family is the fundamental unit of society and the main center for the growth and education of human beings. Compatibility concerning belief and ideal, which provides the primary basis for man's development and growth, is the main consideration in the establishment of a family. The Islamic government must provide the necessary facilities for the attainment of this goal. This view of the family unit prevents women from being regarded as an object or as an instrument in the service of promoting consumerism and exploitation. Not only does woman recover thereby her momentous and precious function of motherhood, rearing of ideologically committed human beings, but she also assumes a pioneering social role and becomes the fellow struggler of man in all vital areas of life. Given the weighty responsibilities that woman thus assumes, she is accorded in Islam great value and nobility."

"12. The planning of a correct and just economic system, by Islamic criteria, to create welfare, eliminate poverty, and abolish all forms of deprivation concerning food, housing, work, health care, and the provision of social insurance for all.

Rights of children

Inalienable rights Human dignity

Right to own property Right to life

Freedom of opinion/thought/conscience

Freedom of press

Right to privacy Freedom of press

Freedom of association

Right to join trade unions Right to form political parties Restrictions on political parties

Freedom of assembly.

Article 20

All citizens of the country, both men and women, equally enjoy the protection of the law and enjoy all human, political, economic, social, and cultural rights, in conformity with Islamic criteria.'

Article 21

The government must ensure the rights of women in all respects, in conformity with Islamic criteria, and accomplish the following goals:

1. create a favorable environment for the growth of women's personalities and the restoration of their rights, both material and intellectual.

2. the protection of mothers, particularly during pregnancy and childrearing, and the protection of children without guardians.

3. establishing competent courts to protect and preserve the family.

4. the provision of special insurance for widows, and aged women and women

without support.

5. the awarding of guardianship of children to worthy mothers, to protect the interests of the children, in the absence of a legal guardian."

Article 29

To benefit from social security concerning retirement, unemployment, old age, disability, absence of a guardian, and benefits relating to being stranded, accidents, health services, and medical care and treatment, provided through insurance or other means, is accepted as a universal right.

The government must provide the foregoing services and financial support for every individual citizen by drawing, by the law, on the national revenues and funds obtained through public contributions."

Islamic Republic Healthcare Projects, Programs, and Policies:

There is no centralized accumulation of policies but rather a non-focused and non-centralized piece meals information which do not cover the healthcare systems in a dynamic, progressive amenable to stepwise advancement (personal communications)

There are significant dichotomy between the current status, availability, accessibility, and affordability of healthcare systems and management and transparency of information within the country and published criteria and policy for international feed.

Published in foreign news and online:

What are the main principles of healthcare ethics in Islam?

Each of the four principles (beneficence, nonmaleficence, justice, and autonomy) is investigated in turn, looking at the extent to which each is rooted in the Islamic paradigm.

how does Islam view healthcare?

Since good health is a gift from God, Muslims believe that taking care of one's health is a religious duty. However, this also implies that Muslims often prefer spiritual well-being over physical wellness. Religious beliefs may also influence a Muslim patient's notions of healing (4, 2022)

What is the health system structure of Iran?

... Iran's health system follows a hierarchical referral network, and its services to the community are provided in the form of PHC. In this structure, comprehensive urban and rural health centers are responsible for delivering health services to the people of a specific region [13].

The Islamic Republic of Iran (Iran) is a great country with a wide area and dispersed population. You may find only a few countries in the world that neighbor 17 countries two of them are involved in a concurring war. The weather, culture, environmental hazards the infrastructures, and ultimately heath indicators have a great diversity in Iran. The specific geographic situation of Iran's mass immigration from Afghanistan and Iraq, the wars and insecurity after it in the region, and illegal drug traffic from eastern borders with Pakistan and Afghanistan have all affected the health system in Iran (1).

There are noticeable health inequalities within the country; for instance, the difference in life expectancy between different provinces reaches 24 years. The same is through for almost all indicators excluding the vaccine coverage and access to primary health care which are above 90% nationwide.

While the major burden of disease in the country as a whole and especially in the large metropolitans is noncommunicable diseases (NCDs) including cardiovascular disease (CVD), cancer, and injuries, the country is still faced with the problem of infectious diseases which in many instances are somehow related to its neighbor countries (2, 3). In both recent epidemics of Cholera which occurred in Iran in 2005 and 2007 through fingerprinting of the bacteria, it was clearly shown that organisms were imported from Pakistan and Iraq respectively (4). Crimean Congo fever previously not known in Iran is now a real health hazard with up to 250 cases each year affected with a fatality rate of 25%. All these reported cases were related to smuggled poultry from neighboring countries. Two out of four countries that could not still eradicate poliomyelitis are neighbors of Iran. Despite these challenges, it is now 12 years that Iran has obtained the certificate of polio eradication and sustained this success. Malaria although previously endemic in Iran is now confined to three southeastern provinces with the majority of falciparum cases being foreigners who entered the country illegally.

These threats could not stop the success of the Ministry of Health and Medical Education (HOME) in control of all epidemics and even in helping the neighboring countries through the so-called Group 5 initiative which was launched in 2005 during the Eastern Mediterranean regional meeting of the world health organization (WHO) between Iran, Iraq, Pakistan, Afghanistan, and WHO with the central role of Iran as the secretary. This could

have been done only through strengthening primary health care (PHC), active surveillance and frequent monitoring, vaccination at borders and even sending free vaccines to the neighboring countries.

Working for the future is based on our current capacities. This is through analyzing the previous achievements realizing today's needs and predicting fluctuating situations in tomorrow. In this study, we reviewed some of the achievements of the Iranian health system in recent decades.

Integration of Medical Education and Service Provision Iran has applied the principles of Alma Ata but this was not just like rewriting a written statement; Iran has had its model. Integration of medical education and health services and accountability of the educational system to match the real needs of the population have changed our situation from a country hosting more than 3000 working foreign physicians in 1983 to a country fulfilling all her needs in higher education in the health and medical sciences (5). The expansion of medical education while the country was suffering from an imposed war that lasted 8 years and while confronting a sanction lasting now for more than 29 years is a unique experiment in the world. You may see such an expansion in other countries, but this usually happens through foreign support. For the health workers or as is called in Iran Behvarz, the initial group was based on those rural inhabitants who completed their elementary educations. They then entered the special training program for 2 years and then appointed as Behvarz to the health house covering up to 1500 people. The major strength of the administration process was introducing the most appropriate local people to local health authorities by rural councils for being a Behavrz. This resulted in a proper environment that helped the health system to have the support of the community. Only through this support, it was possible to improve the health indicators dramatically during a very short period. For instance, it took only 3 years to increase neonatal vaccine coverage from 33% to over 90% nationwide (6).

Although continuous professional development programs for all of them were conducted and they became experienced and educated further they had only elementary education. The health system initiatives had to be tailored so that these 30,000 Behvarzes as the main acting boa dies could be participated [6]. The reason for choosing the vital horoscope as a simple model of the census has turned the Behavrzy into a university degree. Although the central role of people in appointing the Behvarz has been maintained, they are now appointed from those rural inhabitants who have successively graduated from high schools. This promotion in Behvarz activity now has increased the capacity of the health system and more sophisticated health programs could become a reality. For instance, screening for diabetes and hypertension now covers almost all inhabitants of cities with less than 20,000 population and all rural regions. Interestingly using HBA1c as an indicator of blood sugar control it was shown that known diabetic patients of this group have a better control of their blood sugar compared to urban inhabitants (7, 8).

"According to the WHO as of 2000, Iran ranks 58 in healthcare and 93 in health system performance. In 2016 Bloomberg News ranked Iran's 30th most efficient healthcare system ahead of the United States and Brazil. The report shows life expectancy in Iran is 75.5 years and per capita spending on healthcare is $346. The health status of Iranians has improved over the last two decades, Iran has been able to extend public health preventive services through the establishment of a primary care network. As a result, child and maternal mortality rates have fallen significantly, and life expectancy at birth has risen remarkably."

I have communicated this information to more than 50 physicians with different specialties working in many different settings and institutions and cannot verify any of the mentioned claims, yet the response and reports are opposite and heartbreaking (personal communications)

It appears that all aspects of the healthcare system, preventive care, and medical education are in a state of collapse, predicting a disastrous outcome.

Next step: vision

It is prudent to understand the dichotomy of healthcare reality and fantasy representation by the Islamic Republic and its agents and lobbyists.

Any plan of action should identify the current and true existing healthcare, healthcare management system, policies (if they exist and have even not been implemented), existing infrastructures and workforce, identify the leaders in healthcare, and create a model which best fits the current and existing healthcare system, and establish a functional bridge with 21-century healthcare system which truly service and satisfy the total needs of 80 million Iranian with their needs and expectation.

Islamic Republic of Iran Healthcare systems Weaknesses, failures, and opportunity for improvement Abstract

CONCEPT:

The General Healthcare system is defined by a reductionist perspective phenomenon.

The health system should be viewed as a comprehensive system in terms of its goals, institution supply side of the health system with population as a common denominator.

Healthcare systems are further defined by their functions, equity, responsiveness, expectations, and effective and equitable financing.

PROBLEMS

Iran's health system is a hierarchical referral network in a Primary Healthcare (PHC) structure and has three structural pillars: Public Health, Private sector, and Non- non-governmental organizations (funded by private funds and charitable organizations). The overall Health System is embedded in Islamic mandates and Shariah law in terms of organization, administration, physical plant, and delivery.

FAILURES

There are significant and noticeable discrepancies in reporting and lack of transparency and false reporting by the IR government and even some representatives affiliated with international organizations, such as UNICEF which could not be verified (personal communications)

There are close to 900 hospitals, 75% of those in urban areas and major cities 25% in rural and small cities, and almost none in hard-to-reach areas.

At least 75% of Iran's population lives in urban areas and cities and 25% in rural andremote areas with scarce resources and a lack of functional delivery systems.

Index Mundi reports 1.56 hospital beds per 1000 people.IR reports 1.2hospital per 100000 people. Even those statistics could not be verified (personal communications).

LESSONS LEARNED:

Overall the health system in Iran is underfunded, mismanaged, and in many areas corrupt.

The payer system is fee-for-service with huge discrepancies in tariffs in urban and rural

areas
which leads to practitioners' dissatisfaction and underperformance and eventually collapse of the system and distrust.

Iran spends 4.1% of the country's GPD on healthcare and, interestingly, the government usually borrows billions of Rials from healthcare rendering the system penniless and accelerating the system's failure. The World Health Organization reported the following deficiencies for five consecutive years.

"• Partially functioning referral system between primary health care facilities and hospitals

• Weak data collection and analysis from the private sector

• Regulations and oversight of the private sector are limited

• The current provider payment method is based on fee for services, which is because of induced demands.

• Share of out-of-pocket payment is high in outpatient services and there is limited information on regulation and oversight mechanisms.

• Difficult to address and investigate the main roots of out-of-pocket expenditure by the patients.

Lack of transparency in allocated resources strategic purchasing and government expenditure.

• Information on quality of health care and consumer satisfaction is not available or is not complete.

• There is an income gap between private and public providers even at different levels in the same group.

• Unregulated tariffs and preferential payment schedules.

• The rationale of benefits package development is not based on scientific principles.

• Lack of information in the area of efficiency and effectiveness and the causes of resource waste.

• Lack of transparency in fiscal responsibilities and budgeting and regularly reviewing and adjusting financial plans for the continuity of the healthcare system. Reform and insufficient share

Lack of continuity in healthcare reform and allocation of resources and contribution to healthcare financing as committed earlier"(WHO report , East Mediterranean Region).

OPPORTUNITIES & PLAN OF ACTION DURING TRANSITIONAL GOVERNMENT

A FRAMEWORK FOR LONG-TERM REBUILDING THE HEALTH SYSTEMS:

The healthcare system in Iran is at its nadir from its modern inception, underperforming with profoundly dissatisfied healthcare providers at all levels, and dissatisfied and hopeless patients with increased morbidity and mortality in both primary and secondary prevention and therapeutic medicine.

Actionable proposals:

1- Increase awareness and readiness of the healthcare providers to accept new changes and buy, from new perspectives.

2- Historically the private network is well-developed efficient and widespread. With organized and comprehensive interventions and empowering the regional and local leaders, healthcare revitalization become a reality in a short period.

3- Historically Iran's healthcare systems were founded based on decentralized philosophy. This structure provides ample opportunities to start remedial interventions at different levels, based on local needs, and create independent centers with opportunities for expansion and interrelating models with other centers for wider coverage in all aspects of inpatient and outpatient care.

4- Create strong medical education with a solid and rich foundation currently in the dormant phase of their existence, ready to take over a new role not only in medical education but in the delivery of care.

5- Strong primary care network, amenable to retraining, updating, and restructuring to a modern primary care system.

6- strong and highly educated and technically skilled workforce outside the country and committed to engaging in the modern revitalization of Iran's health system.

Iran Diasporas

Opposition Groups and Organizations:

Several Iranian opposition groups in America oppose the Islamic Republic of Iran. Some prominent ones include the National Council of Resistance of Iran (NCRI), the Mojahedin-e Khalq (MEK), and the Iranian American Community of Northern California (IACNC). These groups advocate for regime change in Iran and support the Iranian people's struggle for democracy, human rights, and freedom. They often organize protests, conferences, and other activities to raise awareness about the human rights abuses and political repression in Iran. Some other opposition groups are considered.

"thinktank" "thought Leaders" and collectively consist of Professionals, academicians (technocrats), writers, and politicians. Other than MEK, all advocate regimes change through political processes and dialogs.

Some of the common advocacies include:

1. Regime Change: These groups seek the overthrow of the current regime in Iran, the Islamic Republic, and aspire to establish a democratic government that respects human rights, freedom of expression, and the rule of law.
2. Democracy and Human Rights: They advocate for the establishment of a democratic system in Iran where the Iranian people can freely elect their leaders and have a say in the governance of the country. They also emphasize the need for protecting and promoting human rights, including freedom of speech, assembly, and religion.
3. Women's Rights: Iranian opposition groups often prioritize women's rights and gender equality. They aim to eliminate discriminatory laws and practices against women and promote equal opportunities and rights for women in all spheres of life.
4. Nuclear Program and Regional Influence: These groups oppose Iran's nuclear program and its regional influence, which they believe poses a threat to regional stability and international security. They call for a peaceful and non-nuclear Iran that respects the sovereignty of its neighboring countries.
5. Support for Protests and Opposition Movements: Iranian opposition groups actively support and encourage protests and opposition movements within Iran. They provide platforms for Iranian activists to raise their voices and advocate for change, both domestically and internationally.
6. It's important to note that different opposition groups may have varying priorities and specific focus and approach.

It's also important to note that despite the growing number of opposition groups in the past 44 years since the Islamic Revolution, their collective and selective advocacies and actions have not borne any fruit or effectively supported the inside Iran opposition groups.

Reviewing the Iranian struggles, protests brutal suppression, and massacre, dictate more presence and specific subversives undertaking.

Who Are Technocrats?

Technocrats are individuals who advocate for or hold positions of power based on their technical expertise and knowledge rather than political or ideological affiliations. They are often professionals in fields such as science, technology, engineering, and economics.

Technocrats believe that decision-making should be guided by scientific and technical considerations rather than political or popular opinion. They argue that expertise and evidence-based approaches should be the primary drivers of policymaking, as they believe that technical knowledge and efficiency can lead to effective governance and problem-solving.

Technocrats often promote meritocracy, where individuals are appointed or elected based on their qualifications and expertise rather than political connections or popularity. They may advocate for policies that prioritize data-driven decision-making, efficiency, and expertise to address complex societal challenges.

However, the rise of technocrats in governance can also raise concerns. Critics argue that technocracy may undervalue democratic principles, as it may concentrate power in the hands of a few experts and limit public participation and accountability. Additionally, the technocratic approach may overlook social and ethical considerations, as it tends to prioritize technical solutions over broader societal implications.

Technocrats believe that decisions should be based on data, analysis, and the expertise of professionals in relevant fields. They emphasize the importance of using scientific methods, research, and empirical evidence to inform policy choices. Technocrats argue that this approach can lead to more effective and efficient governance, as decisions are made based on objective information and expertise.

The belief in evidence-based decision-making is rooted in the idea that technical knowledge and expertise can help address complex societal challenges systematically and rationally. Technocrats often advocate for policies that prioritize data-driven decision-making, efficiency, and expertise, as they believe these factors can lead to better outcomes for society.

However, it is important to note that the rise of technocrats in governance can also raise concerns. Critics argue that technocracy may undervalue democratic principles, as it may concentrate power in the hands of a few experts and limit public participation and accountability. Additionally, the technocratic approach may overlook social and ethical considerations, as it tends to prioritize technical solutions over broader societal implications.

Overall, technocrats are individuals who prioritize technical expertise and evidence-based approaches in decision-making, often advocating for policies that prioritize efficiency and expertise in addressing complex societal challenges.

The main belief of technocrats when it comes to decision-making is that it should be guided by scientific and technical considerations rather than political or popular opinion. Technocrats argue that expertise and evidence-based approaches should be the primary drivers of policymaking.

Fighting Corruption.

The role of technocrats in fighting a corrupt government can be significant. Technocrats, with their expertise, knowledge, and commitment to rational decision-making, can play a crucial role in addressing corruption and promoting good governance. Here are some ways in which technocrats can contribute:

1. Transparency and Accountability: Technocrats can advocate for greater transparency and accountability in government processes and operations. They can promote the use of technology and data-driven systems to reduce opportunities for corruption and enhance transparency in decision-making.
2. Strengthening Institutions: Technocrats can work towards strengthening institutions responsible for combating corruption, such as anti-corruption agencies, auditing bodies, and judicial systems. They can contribute their expertise in designing and implementing effective anti-corruption measures and reforms.
3. Policy Reforms: Technocrats can identify and propose policy reforms aimed at reducing corruption and improving governance. They can analyze existing policies, identify loopholes, and suggest changes to enhance transparency, accountability, and integrity in government operations.
4. Capacity Building: Technocrats can contribute to capacity-building efforts by providing training and support to government officials and civil servants. By sharing their expertise and knowledge, they can help build a more professional and competent bureaucracy, less prone to corruption.
5. Advocacy and Awareness: Technocrats can engage in advocacy and awareness campaigns to highlight the negative impacts of corruption and the importance of good governance. They can collaborate with civil society organizations, media, and other stakeholders to raise public awareness and mobilize support for anti-corruption efforts.
6. International Cooperation: Technocrats can participate in international forums and collaborate with international organizations to share best practices, learn from successful anti-corruption initiatives, and seek support for their efforts in fighting corruption.

However, it is important to recognize that technocrats alone cannot eliminate corruption. Addressing corruption requires a comprehensive approach involving political will, strong legal frameworks, public participation, and an engaged civil society. Technocrats can act as catalysts and provide valuable expertise, but sustained efforts from all sectors of society are essential for effectively fighting corruption in a government.

Technocrats and Technology.

Technocrats can utilize technology and innovation to enhance transparency and accountability in governance in the following ways:

1. Open Data Platforms: Technocrats can advocate for the establishment of open data platforms that provide easy access to government information, budgets, expenditures, and procurement processes. By making data readily available to the public, citizens and civil society organizations can hold governments accountable and monitor the use of public resources.
2. E-Governance Solutions: Technocrats can promote the adoption of e-governance solutions to streamline government processes and reduce opportunities for corruption. This includes implementing online portals for citizen services, digital platforms for government transactions, and electronic documentation systems that minimize human intervention and potential manipulation.
3. Blockchain Technology: Technocrats can explore the use of blockchain technology to enhance transparency and accountability in governance. Blockchain provides a decentralized and tamper-proof system for recording and verifying transactions, making it difficult for corruption to go unnoticed. It can be applied to areas such as land registration, procurement, and financial transactions.
4. Digital Identity Systems: Technocrats can advocate for the implementation of digital identity systems that ensure the uniqueness and authenticity of individuals. These systems can help prevent identity fraud and facilitate efficient and transparent service delivery, reducing the potential for corruption in public administration.
5. Data Analytics: Technocrats can leverage data analytics techniques to analyze large volumes of data and detect patterns of corruption. By analyzing government expenditures, financial transactions, and procurement processes, they can identify irregularities, anomalies, and potential instances of corruption that may otherwise go unnoticed.
6. Whistleblower Platforms: Technocrats can support the development of secure and anonymous whistleblower platforms that allow individuals to report corruption and wrongdoing without fear of retaliation. These platforms can facilitate the collection of evidence and enable authorities to take appropriate action against corrupt practices.
7. Social Media and Citizen Engagement: Technocrats can utilize social media platforms and digital tools to engage citizens and encourage their active participation in governance processes. By leveraging technology, they can promote public consultation, gather feedback, and enable citizens to report corruption incidents in

real-time.

8. Data Visualization and Dashboards: Technocrats can develop data visualization tools and dashboards that present complex government data in a user-friendly and understandable format. These visualizations can help citizens, journalists, and civil society organizations comprehend and analyze information related to government performance, budgets, and expenditures.

By harnessing the power of technology and innovation, technocrats can create systems and tools that promote transparency, accountability, and citizen participation in governance. These advancements can help prevent corruption, improve service delivery, and build trust between governments and their citizens.

Blockchain Technology.

Blockchain technology plays a significant role in promoting transparency and accountability in governance by providing a decentralized and tamper-proof system for recording and verifying transactions. Here are some key ways in which blockchain technology can enhance transparency and accountability:

1. Immutable Record-Keeping: Blockchain technology enables the creation of a transparent and immutable record of transactions. Once a transaction is recorded on the blockchain, it cannot be altered or deleted, ensuring the integrity of the data. This feature makes it difficult for corrupt practices to go unnoticed and allows for easy verification of transactions.

2. Eliminating Intermediaries: By leveraging blockchain technology, governments can reduce the need for intermediaries in various processes. This eliminates the potential for corruption and manipulation by removing the central authority that traditionally controls and verifies transactions. Instead, transactions are verified by the decentralized network of participants, ensuring transparency and reducing the risk of corruption.

3. Smart Contracts: Blockchain allows for the implementation of smart contracts, which are self-executing agreements with predefined rules and conditions. These contracts are automatically enforced and executed when the predetermined conditions are met, eliminating the need for intermediaries and reducing the potential for corruption or manipulation.

4. Enhanced Security: Blockchain technology provides a high level of security through cryptographic encryption and consensus mechanisms. This ensures that transactions and data stored on the blockchain are protected from unauthorized access and tampering. By securing sensitive government information and transactions, blockchain technology helps to prevent corruption and fraudulent activities.

5. Public Auditing and Accountability: The transparency of blockchain allows for public auditing and accountability. All transactions recorded on the blockchain are

visible to all participants, making it easier to track and monitor the flow of funds and resources. This transparency enables citizens, civil society organizations, and auditors to verify government expenditures, budgets, and procurement processes, holding governments accountable for their actions.

6. Traceability and Supply Chain Management: Blockchain technology can be utilized to track and trace the movement of goods and resources throughout the supply chain. This transparency ensures that there is no tampering, counterfeiting, or diversion of resources, enhancing accountability and preventing corruption in procurement processes.
7. Whistleblower Protection: Blockchain technology can provide a secure and anonymous platform for whistleblowers to report corruption and wrongdoing. By leveraging blockchain's encryption and decentralized nature, individuals can safely report instances of corruption without fear of retaliation, ensuring the protection of whistleblowers and facilitating the investigation of corrupt practices.
8. Decentralization: Blockchain operates on a decentralized network of computers called nodes. Transactions are recorded and verified by multiple nodes, and a consensus mechanism ensures that all participants agree on the validity of transactions. This decentralization prevents a single entity or authority from having control over the transaction process, reducing the risk of corruption and manipulation.
9. Immutable Ledger: Once a transaction is recorded on the blockchain, it becomes a permanent part of the ledger and cannot be altered or deleted. Each block in the blockchain contains a cryptographic hash, which is a unique identifier that links it to the previous block. This chain of linked blocks creates an immutable record of transactions, making it extremely difficult for anyone to manipulate or tamper with the data.
10. Transparency: Blockchain provides transparency by allowing all participants on the network to have access to the same information. Every transaction recorded on the blockchain is visible to all participants, ensuring that any suspicious activity can be easily detected and investigated. This transparency acts as a deterrent to corruption because it becomes much harder to engage in illicit activities without being noticed.
11. Consensus Mechanisms: Blockchain uses consensus mechanisms, such as Proof of Work (PoW) or Proof of Stake (PoS), to validate and verify transactions. These mechanisms require participants to solve complex mathematical problems or stake their cryptocurrency to validate transactions. This consensus process ensures that transactions are verified by multiple participants and prevents a single individual or group from manipulating the transaction records.
12. Smart Contracts: Smart contracts are self-executing agreements with predefined rules and conditions. They are automatically enforced and executed on the

blockchain when the specified conditions are met. By eliminating the need for intermediaries and relying on predefined rules, smart contracts reduce the potential for corruption and manipulation in contractual agreements.

13. Encryption and Security: Blockchain technology uses cryptographic encryption to secure transactions and data. Each transaction is encrypted and linked to the previous transaction using cryptographic hashes, ensuring the integrity and security of the data. This encryption makes it extremely difficult for hackers or malicious actors to tamper with the transactions or manipulate the data.

Overall, blockchain technology offers a powerful tool for promoting transparency and accountability in governance by providing a secure, transparent, and tamper-proof infrastructure for recording and verifying transactions. It has the potential to revolutionize traditional governance systems, reduce corruption, and enhance public trust in government institutions.

Decentralization Concept.

Decentralization in blockchain technology plays a crucial role in preventing corruption and manipulation in transactions. Here's how:

1. No Single Point of Control: In a decentralized blockchain network, there is no single point of control or authority. Transactions are verified and recorded by multiple nodes spread across the network. This eliminates the risk of a single entity having control over the transaction process, reducing the potential for corruption or manipulation by a central authority.
2. Consensus Mechanism: Decentralized blockchain networks rely on consensus mechanisms, such as Proof of Work (PoW) or Proof of Stake (PoS), to validate transactions. These mechanisms require participants to contribute computational power or stake their cryptocurrency to validate transactions. Consensus is reached when a majority of participants agree on the validity of a transaction. This distributed consensus process ensures that transactions are validated by multiple participants, making it difficult for any single entity to manipulate the transaction records.
3. Transparency and Audibility: Decentralized blockchains provide transparency by allowing all participants to have access to the same information. Every transaction recorded on the blockchain is visible to all participants, making it easier to detect any suspicious activity. The transparency and audibility of the blockchain make it challenging for corrupt practices to go unnoticed, as any attempt to manipulate the transactions would be visible to the entire network.
4. Trust through Verification: Decentralization in blockchain technology promotes trust through verification. As transactions are verified by multiple nodes in the network, participants can trust the integrity and validity of the transactions without

relying on a central authority. This trust in the decentralized verification process reduces the potential for corruption and manipulation, as participants have confidence in the transparency and reliability of the blockchain system.

5. Immutable Ledger: Blockchain's decentralized nature ensures that once a transaction is recorded on the blockchain, it becomes a permanent part of the ledger and cannot be altered or deleted. Each block in the blockchain contains a cryptographic hash that links it to the previous block, creating an immutable record of transactions. This immutability makes it extremely difficult for any individual or entity to manipulate the transaction history without the consensus of the network.

By eliminating the need for a central authority, promoting transparency, relying on consensus mechanisms, and ensuring an immutable ledger, decentralization in blockchain technology significantly reduces the potential for corruption and manipulation in transactions. It creates a system where trust is built upon verifiable and transparent processes, making it challenging for dishonest actors to exploit the system for their gain.

The main difference between Proof of Stake (PoS) and Delegated Proof of Stake (DPoS) consensus mechanisms lies in the way validators are selected and the role they play in the network. Here are the key distinctions:

1. Validator Selection:

- PoS: In a Proof of Stake system, validators are chosen based on the number of coins they hold and are willing to "stake" as collateral. The more coins a validator has, the higher their chances of being chosen to validate transactions and create new blocks.

- DPoS: Delegated Proof of Stake introduces an additional layer of selection. Instead of all participants being eligible to become validators, the network's participants vote to select a limited number of delegates from a pool of candidates. These delegates, also known as block producers or witnesses, are responsible for validating transactions and creating new blocks.

2. Role of Validators:

- PoS: In a PoS system, validators take turns to validate transactions and create new blocks based on their stake in the network. The selection of validators is usually random or based on a combination of factors such as the amount of stake and the length of time the coins have been held.

- DPoS: In DPoS, the elected delegates have a more active role in the network. They are responsible for validating transactions and producing new blocks continuously. The number of delegates is typically limited, which allows for faster block confirmation times and higher transaction throughput compared to PoS.

3. Consensus Process:

- PoS: In Proof of Stake, validators independently validate transactions and propose new blocks. Once a validator has validated a block, they broadcast it to the network, and other validators verify its correctness before accepting it.

- DPoS: In Delegated Proof of Stake, the selected delegates are responsible for validating transactions and producing new blocks collectively. They take turns in a predetermined order, with each delegate having a fixed time slot to propose a block. This process reduces the number of rounds of communication required for consensus and speeds up block production.

4. Governance and Scalability:

- PoS: Proof of Stake systems typically have a more decentralized governance structure, as validators are selected based on their stake. However, the scalability of PoS networks can be limited due to the computational requirements of validating transactions for all participants.

- DPoS: Delegated Proof of Stake introduces a more centralized governance structure, as the selection of delegates is based on voting. This allows for faster block confirmation times and higher transaction throughput, making DPoS networks more scalable.

Both PoS and DPoS are consensus mechanisms designed to achieve consensus in decentralized blockchain networks, but DPoS introduces a more efficient and scalable approach by delegating the block production responsibility to a limited number of elected delegates. The choice between PoS and DPoS depends on factors such as network goals, decentralization requirements, scalability needs, and the level of trust among participants.

Technocrats and Advocacy Groups Roles and Mandates:

The current opposition groups outside Iran must transform from advocacy opposition to more actionable groups and seek internal and foreign support to bring about more tangible subversive results.

Technocrats, who are highly skilled professionals in their respective fields, can potentially play a role in subverting a corrupt government. While their effectiveness may vary depending on the specific context and challenges, here are some ways in which technocrats can contribute:

1. Expertise and Analysis: Technocrats can provide objective analysis and expertise in areas such as economics, governance, law, and technology. Their knowledge and insights can help identify and expose corruption, inefficiencies, and abuses of power within the government. By providing evidence-based assessments, technocrats can contribute to public discourse and raise awareness about the need for change.
2. Policy Development: Technocrats can contribute to the development of alternative policies and reforms that prioritize transparency, accountability, and good governance. Their expertise can help design and implement policies that address systemic issues and promote ethical practices. By offering viable alternatives, technocrats can

challenge and undermine the corrupt practices of the government.

3. Anti-Corruption Initiatives: Technocrats can lead or support anti-corruption initiatives by utilizing their skills and knowledge to develop strategies, systems, and tools to prevent and detect corruption. This can involve implementing transparent procurement processes, strengthening financial management systems, and promoting whistleblower protection mechanisms. Technocrats can also advocate for the adoption of international standards and best practices in combating corruption.
4. Digital Tools and Innovation: Technocrats can leverage technology and innovation to expose and combat corruption. They can develop digital platforms, data analytics tools, and anti-corruption software to enhance transparency, facilitate citizen engagement, and monitor government activities. By harnessing the power of technology, technocrats can provide citizens with access to information and empower them to hold the government accountable.
5. International Engagement: Technocrats can engage with the international community to seek support, resources, and expertise in combating corruption. They can collaborate with international organizations, participate in anti-corruption networks, and advocate for international cooperation against corrupt governments. This can provide additional leverage and visibility to their efforts.

Building alternative institutions is an important strategy to fight against a dictatorship. These institutions can provide alternative avenues for governance, promote democratic values, and challenge the authoritarian regime. Here are some ways to build alternative institutions:

1. Independent Media: Establishing independent media outlets is crucial for providing accurate and unbiased information to the public. These outlets can expose the regime's propaganda, disseminate news, and foster critical thinking. Support for independent journalism can include funding, training, and legal protection for journalists.
2. Civil Society Organizations: Strengthening civil society organizations, such as human rights groups, advocacy organizations, and grassroots movements, is essential. These organizations can mobilize and empower citizens, monitor the government's actions, and provide platforms for public participation. Support can include capacity building, networking, and funding.
3. Education and Research Institutions: Investing in education and research institutions helps cultivate a culture of critical thinking, knowledge, and innovation. These institutions can promote democratic values, human rights education, and research on governance alternatives. Support can include scholarships, curriculum development, and academic freedom protection.
4. Judicial and Legal Institutions: Building and reinforcing independent and impartial judicial systems is crucial to ensure the rule of law and accountability. Support can include training for judges and lawyers, legal aid programs, and advocacy for judicial independence.

5. Electoral and Political Institutions: Strengthening electoral systems and political parties can provide avenues for democratic transitions. Support can include voter education, election monitoring, and capacity building for political parties committed to democratic principles.
6. Economic Institutions: Developing and promoting inclusive economic institutions can create opportunities for economic growth, reduce corruption, and alleviate poverty. Support can include entrepreneurship programs, microfinance initiatives, and fair trade practices.
7. International Alliances and Support: Building alliances with international organizations, democratic governments, and civil society groups can provide diplomatic and financial support. These alliances can amplify the voice of the opposition, exert pressure on the dictatorship, and provide resources for building alternative institutions.
8. Transitional Justice Mechanisms: Establishing mechanisms for transitional justice, such as truth commissions or special courts, can address past human rights abuses and promote reconciliation. These mechanisms can help restore trust and accountability in society.
9. Digital and Technology Platforms: Leveraging digital and technology platforms can facilitate communication, mobilization, and information dissemination. Online platforms can be used for organizing protests, sharing stories, and circumventing censorship.

Other Building Alternatives;

1. Networking and Collaboration: Foster collaboration among like-minded individuals and organizations. Create networks, alliances, and coalitions to pool resources, share knowledge, and amplify collective efforts. Collaborative initiatives can include joint advocacy campaigns, information sharing platforms, and coordinated actions.
2. Grassroots Movements: Mobilize and empower grassroots movements to challenge the regime's authority. Organize peaceful protests, demonstrations, and civil disobedience actions to raise awareness, build momentum, and demonstrate unity against the dictatorship. Grassroots movements can also engage in community organizing, education, and outreach to empower individuals and foster a sense of collective resistance.
3. Civic Education and Awareness: Promote civic education programs to raise awareness about democratic values, human rights, and the dangers of dictatorship. Develop educational materials, workshops, and training programs to empower citizens with knowledge and critical thinking skills. This can help create an informed and engaged citizenry that actively participates in the fight against the dictatorship.
4. Alternative Media: Establish alternative media platforms such as independent newspapers, radio stations, and online outlets. These platforms can provide accurate

and unbiased information, counter regime propaganda, and amplify the voices of dissent. Support alternative media through funding, training, and legal protection to ensure their sustainability and reach.

5. Parallel Institutions: Create parallel institutions that provide services and support to the community, challenging the regime's monopoly. Examples include alternative healthcare clinics, education centers, legal aid services, and community-driven development projects. These institutions not only meet the needs of the people but also demonstrate the viability of alternative governance structures.
6. Economic Initiatives: Support and promote alternative economic initiatives that empower local communities and reduce dependence on the regime. This can include cooperatives, social enterprises, and fair trade practices. By fostering economic independence and resilience, these initiatives weaken the regime's control over the economy.
7. International Support: Seek international support from democratic governments, human rights organizations, and international institutions. Engage in diplomatic efforts to raise awareness about the dictatorship's human rights abuses, seek sanctions or other forms of pressure, and secure funding for building alternative institutions. International solidarity can provide crucial resources and leverage in the fight against the dictatorship.
8. Legal and Judicial Strategies: Utilize legal and judicial strategies to challenge the regime's actions and seek justice. This can involve filing lawsuits, advocating for legal reforms, and supporting human rights defenders. Legal challenges can expose the regime's violations, create legal precedents, and contribute to the erosion of its legitimacy.
9. Transitional Justice Processes: Plan for transitional justice processes that address past human rights abuses and promote reconciliation. Establish truth commissions, memorialization initiatives, and reparations programs to acknowledge victims' experiences, hold perpetrators accountable, and promote healing and reconciliation in society.
10. It is important to adapt these strategies to the specific context and challenges faced in fighting against the dictatorship. Building alternative institutions requires resilience, creativity, and the collective efforts of individuals, organizations, and communities committed to democratic values and human rights.

Building alternative institutions requires long-term commitment, collaboration, and resources. It is essential to ensure the inclusivity, transparency, and accountability of these institutions to gain public trust and effectively challenge the dictatorship.

However, it is important to note that the effectiveness of technocrats in subverting a corrupt government also depends on several factors, including the level of corruption, the political context, the willingness of the government to engage in reform, and the support they receive from civil society, the private sector, and international actors. Additionally, technocrats may face challenges and risks in their efforts, including political resistance, intimidation, and reprisals from the government.

Ultimately, the success of technocrats in subverting a corrupt government relies on their ability to build alliances, mobilize public support, and navigate the complex dynamics of power and politics. Collaboration with civil society organizations, grassroots movements, and other stakeholders is crucial for a comprehensive and sustainable approach to bring about change.

Unwilling to Reform Dictatorship:

Subverting a dictatorship unwilling to reform is an immensely challenging and risky endeavor. Dictatorships are characterized by centralized power, repression, and the absence of democratic institutions. Here are some of the challenges and risks involved in such a situation:

1. Lack of Political Space: Dictatorships tightly control political space, restricting freedom of speech, assembly, and association. Technocrats attempting to subvert such a regime face severe limitations in organizing and mobilizing opposition. The lack of a supportive political environment hampers their ability to openly advocate for reform or mobilize public support.
2. State Surveillance and Repression: Dictatorships employ extensive surveillance apparatuses and suppress dissent through intimidation, arbitrary arrests, torture, or even extrajudicial killings. Technocrats involved in subverting the regime are at high risk of being targeted by state security forces, leading to personal safety concerns for themselves and their associates.
3. Lack of International Support: Subverting a dictatorship without international support can be extremely challenging. Dictators often maintain alliances with powerful countries or have strategic importance, making it difficult to garner meaningful international support for regime change or intervention. Without external assistance, technocrats may struggle to overcome the regime's resources and influence.
4. Disinformation and Propaganda: Dictatorships excel at controlling information flow and manipulating public opinion through state-controlled media and propaganda. Technocrats face the challenge of countering disinformation campaigns that aim to discredit their efforts and maintain the regime's grip on power. Overcoming these propaganda tactics requires strategic communication and building alternative channels for information dissemination.
5. Internal Divisions and Fragmentation: Opposition movements in dictatorships often suffer from internal divisions, rivalries, and fragmentation. Technocrats face the challenge of uniting diverse groups, ideologies, and interests to form a cohesive and effective opposition. Overcoming these divisions and building a unified front is crucial for subverting the regime.

6. Co-optation and Infiltration: Dictatorships may attempt to co-opt or infiltrate opposition movements to neutralize dissent. Technocrats must be vigilant against attempts by the regime to undermine their efforts through coercion, bribery, or infiltration. Maintaining trust, transparency, and security protocols within the movement becomes crucial to protect against internal sabotage.
7. Economic and Social Challenges: Dictatorships often prioritize their own self-interests over the welfare of the population. Technocrats attempting to subvert the regime must navigate economic and social challenges, such as widespread poverty, inequality, and lack of basic services. Addressing these issues and offering viable alternatives to the regime's governance is essential in gaining public support.

Despite these challenges and risks, technocrats and opposition movements can employ various strategies to subvert a dictatorship unwilling to reform. These include building strong grassroots movements, utilizing technology for communication and organizing, engaging in nonviolent resistance, fostering international solidarity, and employing creative tactics to expose and challenge the regime's abuses. It is essential to recognize that subverting a dictatorship requires resilience, strategic planning, and a long-term commitment to bringing about democratic change.

Accepting Risk:

Technocrats face several challenges and risks in their efforts to subvert a corrupt government. Here are some of the common ones:

1. Political Resistance: Technocrats may face significant political resistance from corrupt government officials who benefit from the existing system. These officials may actively obstruct or undermine the efforts of technocrats to expose corruption and implement reforms. Politically powerful individuals or interest groups may use their influence to discredit or marginalize technocrats, making it difficult for them to bring about meaningful change.
2. Intimidation and Reprisals: Technocrats who challenge a corrupt government can face various forms of intimidation and reprisals. They may be subjected to threats, harassment, or even physical harm. Their careers, reputations, and personal safety may be at risk. The fear of retaliation can discourage technocrats from speaking out or pursuing their efforts to subvert corruption.
3. Lack of Institutional Support: Technocrats often face a lack of institutional support within the government itself. Bureaucratic structures and processes may be resistant to change, making it challenging for technocrats to implement reforms or enforce anti-corruption measures. Some technocrats may find themselves isolated or marginalized within their own organizations, making it difficult to gain traction in their efforts.
4. Limited Resources: Technocrats may face constraints in terms of resources, both financial and human. The lack of adequate funding, staffing, and infrastructure can

hinder their ability to effectively investigate corruption, develop and implement reforms, and sustain their initiatives over the long term. Limited resources can also impede their ability to compete with the resources available to corrupt officials.

5. Legal and Regulatory Challenges: Technocrats may encounter legal and regulatory obstacles that hinder their efforts. Corrupt governments may have laws or regulations in place that restrict or criminalize activities aimed at exposing corruption or advocating for reform. Technocrats may face legal threats, lawsuits, or prosecutions as a result of their actions. Navigating the legal landscape can be complex and risky for technocrats.
6. Lack of Public Awareness and Support: Technocrats may struggle to generate public awareness and support for their cause. The public may be unaware of the extent of corruption or apathetic towards the issue. Without public pressure and support, it can be difficult for technocrats to build momentum and bring about meaningful change. Overcoming public indifference or skepticism requires effective communication and engagement strategies.
7. International Constraints: Technocrats may face challenges in obtaining international support or cooperation. Some corrupt governments may have alliances or dependencies with powerful international actors, making it difficult for technocrats to receive assistance or leverage international pressure. Diplomatic considerations, geopolitical dynamics, or economic interests can limit the support available to technocrats from the international community.

Despite these challenges and risks, technocrats who are committed to subverting a corrupt government can find ways to navigate and overcome them. Building alliances with civil society organizations, engaging with the international community, leveraging technology, and mobilizing public support are some strategies that can enhance their effectiveness and resilience.

The Subversion Doctrine, also known as the Doctrine of Subversion, refers to a political strategy or ideology that aims to undermine and weaken an established system or government from within. It involves using various tactics, such as propaganda, disinformation, infiltration, and manipulation, to erode the foundations and legitimacy of the targeted system.

Subversion:

Subversion doctrine is often associated with covert actions, psychological warfare, and unconventional tactics employed by intelligence agencies, revolutionary groups, or ideological movements. It seeks to exploit existing social, political, and economic vulnerabilities to create instability and ultimately facilitate a change in power or the overthrow of the existing regime.

It is important to note that the term "Subversion Doctrine" can have different interpretations and may be used differently in various contexts. In some cases, it may refer to a specific strategy or doctrine followed by a particular organization or state, while in others, it may be a more general concept used to describe subversive activities or tactics employed by various actors.

Overall, the Subversion Doctrine is a complex and controversial topic that involves the manipulation of information, institutions, and public opinion to undermine and weaken established systems of governance.

There are several tactics that can be used in the Subversion Doctrine to undermine and weaken an established system or government. Here are some common tactics:

1. Propaganda: Spreading false or misleading information through various channels, such as media outlets, social media, or grassroots organizations, to shape public opinion and undermine trust in the government or system.
2. Disinformation: Deliberately spreading false or misleading information to create confusion, sow discord, and undermine the credibility of the government or institutions.
3. Infiltration: Sending agents or sympathizers to infiltrate key institutions, organizations, or government agencies to gather intelligence, manipulate decision-making processes, or create internal divisions.
4. Psychological warfare: Using psychological tactics, such as spreading fear, uncertainty, and doubt, to weaken morale, erode trust in leadership, and create a sense of instability within the population.
5. Protests and demonstrations: Organizing and supporting protests, demonstrations, or civil disobedience campaigns to create social unrest, disrupt normal functioning, and challenge the authority and legitimacy of the government.
6. Economic sabotage: Engaging in activities that aim to disrupt or undermine the economy of a country, such as funding anti-government groups, imposing economic sanctions, or engaging in cyberattacks on critical infrastructure.
7. Political manipulation: Exploiting existing political divisions, promoting extremist ideologies, or supporting opposition groups to fragment support for the government and create political instability.
8. Cultural infiltration: Influencing cultural institutions, educational systems, and media outlets to shape public discourse, promote alternative ideologies, and undermine the values and norms of the established system.

It's important to note that these tactics can vary in intensity and form depending on the specific context and objectives of the actors involved in the Subversion Doctrine.

Propaganda can be effectively used to undermine a government or system by shaping public opinion, manipulating information, and creating a negative perception. Here are some ways propaganda can be employed:

1. Manipulating Information: Propaganda disseminates biased or false information to distort the public's understanding of the government or system. This can involve selectively presenting facts, distorting the truth, or presenting information out of context to create a negative narrative.
2. Creating Dissent: Propaganda aims to fuel dissent and undermine public support for the government or system. It may highlight and exaggerate existing grievances, inequalities, or failures of the government, fostering a sense of injustice or dissatisfaction among the population.
3. Portraying the Government as an Enemy: Propaganda can depict the government or system as an oppressive force, using emotional appeals to create fear, anger, or resentment towards those in power. This can be done by emphasizing instances of corruption, abuse of power, or human rights violations.
4. Discrediting Leaders and Institutions: Propaganda often targets leaders and institutions within the government or system, seeking to undermine their credibility and trustworthiness. It may employ personal attacks, character assassination, or unfounded allegations to damage the reputation of key figures or institutions.
5. Polarizing Society: Propaganda can exploit existing social divisions and amplify them to create further discord within society. By promoting extremist ideologies or promoting divisive narratives, it seeks to fragment support for the government and create a sense of instability.
6. Manipulating Media: Propaganda often seeks to control or manipulate media outlets to ensure the dissemination of its messages. This can involve suppressing dissenting voices, promoting biased reporting, or creating alternative media platforms to spread propaganda more effectively.
7. Exploiting Emotions: Propaganda appeals to emotions such as fear, anger, or frustration to manipulate public sentiment. By evoking strong emotional responses, it can influence public opinion and sway individuals against the government or system.
8. Selective Reporting: Propaganda selectively presents information that supports its desired narrative while omitting or downplaying facts that contradict it. This creates a biased perception and distorts the overall understanding of the government or system.
9. Half-Truths and Misinformation: Propaganda often mixes elements of truth with misinformation or exaggeration. By presenting partial truths or distorting facts, it manipulates the public's perception and skews their understanding of the government or system.

10. Emotional Manipulation: Propaganda appeals to emotions such as fear, anger, or sympathy to influence public opinion. It uses emotionally charged language, vivid imagery, and personal stories to create a strong emotional response and cloud rational judgment.
11. Demonization and Dehumanization: Propaganda may employ tactics to vilify or dehumanize individuals or groups associated with the government or system. By portraying them as enemies or threats, it fosters negative perceptions and undermines support for the government or system.
12. Slogans and Catchphrases: Propaganda often relies on catchy slogans, repetitive phrases, and simple messaging to reinforce a desired narrative. By using memorable and easily digestible slogans, it aims to shape public opinion and reinforce specific beliefs or attitudes.
13. False Expertise and Authority: Propaganda may present false experts or individuals with questionable credentials to lend credibility to its messages. By falsely associating the government or system with trusted figures, it seeks to manipulate public trust and perception.
14. Manipulation of Visuals: Propaganda effectively uses visuals such as photographs, videos, or graphics to distort perception. Images can be selectively chosen or manipulated to create a desired impression or evoke specific emotions.
15. Fabrication of Evidence: In some cases, propaganda may fabricate or manipulate evidence to support its claims. This can include forging documents, creating false testimonies, or spreading doctored images or videos.
16. Censorship and Suppression of Dissent: Propaganda often suppresses dissenting voices and alternative viewpoints to maintain control over the narrative. By limiting access to diverse information and silencing opposition, it restricts the public's understanding of the government or system.
17. Awareness of these techniques can help individuals critically evaluate information, seek multiple perspectives, and develop a more nuanced understanding of the government or system. It is crucial to question sources, verify information, and foster media literacy to counter the impact of propaganda.

It is also essential to be critical and discerning when consuming information, especially during times when propaganda is prevalent. Developing media literacy skills and seeking diverse sources of information can help counter the impact of propaganda and promote a more informed understanding of the government or system.

Psychological Warfare:

Psychological warfare is a strategy that aims to influence the thoughts, emotions, attitudes, and behaviors of individuals or groups. It employs various psychological techniques to manipulate perceptions, sow confusion, and shape public opinion. Here are some key aspects of psychological warfare:

1. Propaganda: Propaganda is a central element of psychological warfare. It involves the dissemination of information or ideas, often with a biased or misleading nature, to influence public opinion and manipulate perceptions. As mentioned earlier, propaganda can employ various techniques to distort understanding and shape attitudes towards a particular government, system, or ideology.
2. Deception: Psychological warfare often involves the use of deception to mislead and confuse the target audience. This can include spreading false information, creating fake news, or using disinformation campaigns to undermine trust and sow doubt.
3. Fear and Intimidation: Psychological warfare frequently relies on instilling fear and using intimidation tactics to weaken the morale and resolve of the target population. By creating a sense of insecurity or threat, it aims to manipulate behavior and control the narrative.
4. Psy Ops (Psychological Operations): PsyOps are military activities that utilize psychological warfare techniques to influence the enemy's mindset, morale, and behavior. These operations can involve broadcasting messages, distributing leaflets, or conducting social media campaigns to shape perceptions and attitudes.
5. Perception Management: Psychological warfare seeks to manage and shape public perception through the control of information and narratives. This can involve controlling media outlets, manipulating social media platforms, or using targeted messaging to shape public opinion.
6. Demoralization and Disinformation: Psychological warfare aims to demoralize the enemy by spreading disinformation and undermining their belief systems. This can include attacking their cultural values, spreading rumors, or discrediting their leaders.
7. Psychological Operations in Conflict: In times of armed conflict, psychological warfare is often used to weaken the enemy's morale, undermine their support, and create divisions within their ranks. It can involve tactics such as the dissemination of propaganda, broadcasting psychological messages, or conducting covert operations to influence the enemy's decision-making.

Fear and Risk:

Psychological warfare creates a sense of fear or anxiety in the enemy by using various tactics and techniques. Here are some ways in which it can be achieved:

1. Threats: Psychological warfare may involve issuing direct or indirect threats to instill fear and uncertainty in the enemy. This can be done through public statements, propaganda, or even through intercepted communications.

2. Demonization: Portraying the enemy as dangerous, evil, or inhumane can create fear and anxiety among the population. This can be achieved through propaganda, media manipulation, or spreading rumors and disinformation.
3. Shock and Awe: The use of overwhelming displays of force, such as high-profile military operations or demonstrations, can create a sense of fear and helplessness in the enemy. This can shake their morale and decision-making capabilities.
4. Psychological Operations (PSYOP): PSYOP involves the use of psychological techniques to influence the emotions, beliefs, and behaviors of individuals or groups. This can include the dissemination of frightening images, videos, or messages that evoke fear and anxiety.
5. Targeting Vulnerabilities: Psychological warfare aims to exploit the weaknesses and vulnerabilities of the enemy. By identifying their fears, insecurities, or sensitive issues, psychological warfare can amplify those concerns to create a heightened sense of fear and anxiety.
6. Information Warfare: Spreading false or exaggerated information about potential threats or dangers can create a climate of fear and uncertainty. This can be done through propaganda, disinformation campaigns, or manipulating social media platforms.
7. The objective of creating fear and anxiety is to weaken the morale and decision-making capabilities of the enemy, making them more susceptible to manipulation, demoralization, and ultimately, influencing their actions and outcomes in the conflict.

Psychological Warfare and Techniques.

Portraying the enemy as dangerous or inhumane can create fear and anxiety among the population through several mechanisms:

1. Dehumanization: When the enemy is portrayed as inhumane or subhuman, it becomes easier for people to distance themselves emotionally from them. This dehumanization allows individuals to justify acts of aggression or violence against the enemy, as they are seen as less deserving of empathy or consideration. This perception of the enemy as less than human can generate fear and anxiety among the population, as they may believe that they are facing an enemy that is capable of extreme cruelty or brutality.
2. Threat Perception: By highlighting the perceived dangers posed by the enemy, psychological warfare can manipulate people's perception of the level of threat they face. This can be achieved through propaganda, media manipulation, or exaggerating the enemy's capabilities or intentions. When people believe that they are facing a dangerous and ruthless enemy, it can create a sense of fear and anxiety, leading to a psychological impact on their morale and decision-making.

3. Amplifying Atrocities: Psychological warfare may emphasize or exaggerate real or alleged atrocities committed by the enemy. By highlighting instances of violence, cruelty, or human rights abuses, it can evoke fear and anxiety among the population. The fear of suffering similar atrocities or witnessing loved ones being harmed can weaken morale and decision-making capabilities, as people may become more cautious or hesitant to take action.
4. Spreading Fear through Propaganda: Propaganda can be used to spread fear-inducing messages or imagery about the enemy. This can include depicting the enemy as capable of inflicting great harm, using graphic or disturbing visuals, or creating narratives that emphasize the enemy's destructive power. The repeated exposure to such propaganda can instill a sense of fear and anxiety, leading to a psychological impact on the population.
5. Overall, portraying the enemy as dangerous or inhumane creates fear and anxiety among the population by manipulating their perception of the threat they face and exploiting their emotional responses to dehumanization and fear-inducing tactics. This can weaken morale and decision-making capabilities, making the population more susceptible to manipulation and control.

Aftermath of a revolution

The aftermath of a revolution can be both challenging and overwhelming for a country.

It is a time of great uncertainty and instability, with the potential for both positive and negative outcomes. To navigate this post-revolution period successfully, effective crisis management is essential.

The first step in post-revolution crisis management is to establish a stable government. This may involve creating a new constitution, holding elections, and appointing key officials to key positions. It is important that the government be representative of the people and that its legitimacy be recognized by the international community.

Once a stable government is in place, the next step is to address the immediate needs of the population. This may include providing emergency services such as food, water, and medical care. It may also involve repairing or rebuilding infrastructure such as roads, bridges, and buildings. It is important to prioritize the most urgent needs and to work quickly to address them.

Another key aspect of post-revolution crisis management is to address the underlying causes of the revolution. This may involve addressing issues such as poverty, corruption, and political repression. It may also involve implementing reforms to improve the economy and create jobs. It is important to engage with the population and to listen to their concerns to develop effective solutions.

In addition to these practical measures, it is also important to address the emotional and psychological aftermath of the revolution. Many people may have experienced trauma or loss during the revolution, and it is important to provide support and counseling services to help them heal. It is also important to promote reconciliation and unity within the country and to work to prevent future conflicts.

Finally, it is important to engage with the international community during the post-revolution period. This may involve seeking financial aid and technical assistance to help address the country's needs. It may also involve working to establish positive relationships with neighboring countries and the wider international community.

In conclusion, post-revolution crisis management is a complex and challenging process that requires careful planning, effective leadership, and a commitment to addressing the needs of the population. By working together and taking a strategic approach, it is possible to navigate this challenging period and establish a stable, prosperous, and peaceful future for the country.

In the past 50 years, there have been significant changes in healthcare that have transformed the way medical services are delivered and accessed. Some key changes include:

1. Advancements in technology: The introduction and rapid advancements in medical technology have revolutionized healthcare. From sophisticated imaging techniques like MRI and CT scans to minimally invasive surgical procedures, technology has greatly improved diagnostics, treatment options, and patient outcomes.

2. Electronic health records (EHRs): The digitalization of medical records has streamlined healthcare administration, improved communication between healthcare providers, and enhanced patient safety. EHRs allow for more efficient record-keeping, easy access to patient information, and coordinated care among different healthcare providers.

3. Pharmaceutical advancements: There have been significant advancements in pharmaceuticals, leading to the development of new and more effective drugs. These medications have improved the treatment of many diseases and conditions, extending and enhancing the quality of life for patients.

4. Increased focus on preventive care: In recent years, there has been a shift towards preventive care and wellness promotion. Healthcare providers and policymakers recognize the importance of preventing diseases and promoting healthy lifestyles to reduce healthcare costs and improve overall population health.

5. Expansion of healthcare coverage: The past 50 years have seen various efforts to expand healthcare coverage, particularly in countries like the United States. The implementation of programs like Medicare and Medicaid, as well as the Affordable Care Act (ACA), has increased access to healthcare services for millions of people who were previously uninsured or underinsured.

6. Patient-centered care: Healthcare has shifted towards a more patient-centered approach, focusing on personalized care, shared decision-making, and patient empowerment. Patients are now more involved in their healthcare decisions, and healthcare providers are encouraged to consider patients' preferences and values when providing care.

7. Telemedicine and remote healthcare: The recent advancements in telecommunication technologies have enabled remote healthcare delivery, known as telemedicine. This allows patients to access healthcare services remotely, reducing the need for in-person visits and improving access to care, especially in rural and underserved areas.

These changes have shaped the healthcare landscape and have had a profound impact on patient care, healthcare delivery, and overall health outcomes. However, challenges remain, such as rising healthcare costs, healthcare disparities, and access to care in certain regions.

There are several anticipated physician shortages in various specialties and geographic areas. Some of the main shortages include:

1. Primary care physicians: There is a significant shortage of primary care physicians, who are responsible for providing general medical care and coordinating patient healthcare.

This shortage is expected to worsen as the aging population increases and more people gain access to healthcare through insurance coverage.

2. Specialty physicians: There is also a shortage of specialists in various fields such as cardiology, dermatology, psychiatry, and radiology. These shortages can lead to longer wait times for specialized care and limited access to certain medical services.

3. Rural areas: Rural areas often face more severe physician shortages compared to urban areas. The limited availability of healthcare facilities and the challenges of practicing in remote locations make it difficult to attract and retain physicians in these areas.

4. Geriatrics: With the aging population, there is an anticipated shortage of geriatricians who specialize in the care of elderly patients. This shortage is particularly concerning as the demand for geriatric care is expected to rise significantly in the coming years.

5. Diversity: There is a need for more diversity among physicians to better reflect the diverse patient population. Currently, certain racial and ethnic groups are underrepresented in the physician workforce, leading to disparities in healthcare access and outcomes.

Addressing these anticipated shortages requires various strategies, such as increasing medical school enrollment, expanding residency programs, implementing telemedicine and other technology-based solutions, and offering incentives for physicians to practice in underserved areas.

Geriatric Care:

Geriatric care and the well-being of older Iranians are vastly ignored and underfunded.

One of the best models of care regardless of geography is person-centered, holistic, and carefully individualized.

1- Person-centered care:

This involves recognizing the individuality of each older Iranian, their cultural views, region

And ethnic origin and values.

Elder care is dynamic, and it also involves actively engaging older individuals, their families and

Caregivers. This process will ensure their dignity, privacy, and respect.

2- Holistic care: The care of older people is complex and involves a multi-disciplinary and team Approach. This in addition to managing physical healthcare, but also addressing mental, Emotional, and social well-being.

3- Coordination and integration of care:

This will guarantee seamless care across the healthcare system and different providers.

This will be achieved by implementing care coordinators and care manager teams and

And use of technology to facilitate communications and data sharing.

4- Preventive and early intervention:

This guarantees identifying and addressing health and disease issues early before.

They become more serious, which might need more intensive and costly interventions.

5- Empowerment and self-management:

This involves ensures the involvement of of older person to assume an active

role in managing their health and well-being

This will be achieved through education, coaching, and partnership with healthcare teams.

6- Continuous quality improvement:

This will be achieved by regularly and closely monitoring and reviewing continuously.

Improving the services that have been rendered.

This process will be achieved through partnership with healthcare teams, and feedback by

all. Parties involved, data analysis and benchmarking against best practice models and

Standards.

One of the best models of care for older people ie geriatric population as mentioned above is a "vertical model" of care based on a multidisciplinary team-based approach.

This will be structured as follows:

1- Multidisciplinary team-based care: professionals with different areas of expertise, geriatricians, nurses, pharmacists, social workers, physical therapists, and other providers as needed

2- Comprehensive geriatric assessment: a systemic evaluation of an older person's physical, mental, functional, cognitive, social, and psychological needs.

3- Coordination care: elder care is complex and somehow labor-intensive. Older care needs close and continuous coordination across the providers, hospitals, home, and community.

4-Continuity of care: since older individuals have more complex and multiple health issues and needs, therefore, elder care is ongoing and should be tailored to address changes in health and disease processes.

5- Patient-centered care: this will be achieved by directly involving the patient and family in all decision-making and issues associated with end-of-life issues.

6- family and caregiver support: this is one of the most important components of elder care and
yet mostly underperformed or ignored.

It involves ongoing information sharing and education to familiarize the family with treatment plans and management strategies.

These solutions can help to improve access to quality healthcare services for people living in rural areas in Iran and reduce disparities in healthcare outcomes between urban and rural areas.

Overall, healthcare disparities in Iran are a significant challenge that needs to be addressed through targeted interventions and policies to ensure that all Iranians have equal access to quality healthcare services.

LGBT individuals in Iran face significant healthcare disparities and discrimination. Homosexuality is illegal in Iran and is punishable by imprisonment, flogging, and even death. This has led to a culture of fear and stigma surrounding LGBT individuals, which can prevent them from seeking healthcare services.

LGBT individuals in Iran often face discrimination and mistreatment from healthcare providers, who may view their sexual orientation or gender identity as a moral or religious issue rather than a medical one. This can lead to inadequate or inappropriate healthcare services, as well as a lack of access to necessary treatments and medications.

Transgender individuals in Iran face additional challenges in accessing healthcare, as there are limited options for gender-affirming treatments and surgeries. The legal process for changing one's gender identity is also complex and difficult to navigate, further limiting access to appropriate healthcare services.

Overall, the healthcare disparities faced by LGBT individuals in Iran highlight the urgent need for increased awareness, education, and advocacy to promote inclusive and equitable healthcare services for all.

Healthcare risk assessment after the revolution and transitional period

A healthcare risk assessment after a revolution (during transition) requires a comprehensive approach to identify potential risks. Analyze their impact and develop effective risk mitigation strategies to ensure the health and well-being of the population.

1- Identify the potential Risk:

A healthcare risk includes.

Access to healthcare

Availability of medications and medical supplies Safety of healthcare facilities

Assessment of the impact of political instability on the healthcare systems

2-Analyze the impact of the risks:

Potential impact on healthcare providers

Potential impact on patients

Potential impact on overall population health outcomes and mortality rates

Potential impact on disease prevalence

3-Risk mitigation:

Developing contingency plans for healthcare providers

Ensuring adequate supplies of medications and medical equipment

Implementing measures to stabilize and improve the safety and security of healthcare facilities.

4-Monitor and evaluate the risks and mitigation processes:

Conducting regular risk assessments

Monitoring healthcare outcomes

Evaluating the effectiveness of risk mitigation strategies.

In the immediate aftermath of a revolution in a failed state, healthcare crisis management becomes a crucial aspect of restoring order and providing essential services to the population. Here are some key steps that can be taken:

1. Assess the situation: Conduct a comprehensive assessment of the healthcare system to determine the extent of damage and prioritize areas of immediate concern. Identify critical infrastructure, equipment, and supplies that need urgent attention.

2. Emergency response: Establish emergency medical response teams to address immediate health emergencies and provide medical aid to those injured during the revolution or subsequent unrest. Set up temporary medical facilities, field hospitals, or mobile clinics to ensure access to care.

3. Human resource management: Assess the availability and competency of healthcare professionals. Identify any gaps and develop strategies to rapidly train and mobilize healthcare workers to meet the immediate needs. Encourage local healthcare workers to return to their duties by providing incentives and ensuring their safety.

4. Essential services: Prioritize the provision of essential healthcare services such as emergency care, vaccination programs, maternal and child health services, and

management of communicable diseases. Ensure the availability of medicines, medical supplies, and equipment required to deliver these services.

5. Public health surveillance: Strengthen disease surveillance systems to monitor and respond to any outbreaks or epidemics. Enhance reporting mechanisms for early detection and prevention of communicable diseases. Collaborate with international health organizations to gather resources and expertise.

6. Infrastructure restoration: Repair and rehabilitate damaged healthcare facilities, laboratories, and medical supply chains. Secure access to clean water, electricity, and sanitation facilities to ensure proper infection control measures are in place.

7. Public information: Launch public awareness campaigns to educate the population on health and hygiene practices, prevention of diseases, and the availability of healthcare services. Use various communication channels, including radio, television, and community outreach programs, to disseminate information.

8. Coordination and partnerships: Establish a centralized coordination body involving government authorities, healthcare providers, NGOs, and international organizations to effectively manage the healthcare crisis. Collaborate with humanitarian agencies to secure funding, resources, and technical assistance.

9. Mental health support: Recognize the psychological impact of the revolution and provide mental health support to individuals affected by trauma, violence, or displacement. Develop counseling services and support networks to address mental health issues within the population.

10. Long-term planning: While addressing the immediate crisis, initiate long-term planning for healthcare system reform. Engage local stakeholders, including healthcare professionals, community leaders, and civil society organizations, to design a sustainable and resilient healthcare system that can withstand future challenges.

Overall, in a failed state post-revolution scenario, immediate crisis management of healthcare requires a multi-faceted approach involving emergency response, essential service delivery, infrastructure restoration, coordination, and long-term planning.

Creating a task force, work group, or team for post-revolution crisis management involves assembling a group of individuals with the necessary skills, expertise, and diverse perspectives to address the specific challenges faced. Here are the steps to consider:

1. Define the objectives: Clearly articulate the goals and objectives of the task force, work group, or team. Identify the specific areas or issues that need to be addressed in post-revolution crisis management.

2. Identify key stakeholders: Determine the key stakeholders involved in crisis management, including government officials, healthcare professionals, community leaders, representatives from international organizations, and relevant experts. Ensure representation from different sectors and disciplines to promote comprehensive and

inclusive decision-making.

3. Formulate a structure: Decide on the structure and composition of the task force, work group, or team. Determine the number of members, roles, and responsibilities, and reporting lines. Consider appointing a leader or coordinator who can oversee the activities and ensure smooth functioning.

4. Select members: Identify individuals who possess the necessary expertise, knowledge, and experience relevant to post-revolution crisis management. Seek a diverse range of perspectives, including professionals from the healthcare sector, public administration, finance, logistics, communication, and community engagement. Consider individuals who have experience in crisis management, conflict resolution, and interagency coordination.

5. Establish clear roles and responsibilities: Clearly define the roles and responsibilities of each member within the task force, work group, or team. Assign specific tasks and areas of focus to leverage their expertise effectively. Ensure that everyone understands their responsibilities and the overall objectives of the group.

6. Develop a work plan: Collaboratively develop a work plan that outlines the specific activities, timelines, and deliverables for the task force, work group, or team. Break down the objectives into actionable steps and allocate resources accordingly. Regularly review and update the work plan as needed.

7. Communication and coordination: Establish effective communication channels and mechanisms to facilitate collaboration and coordination within the task force, workgroup, or team. This may include regular meetings, email updates, shared document repositories, and online collaboration tools. Foster an environment that encourages open and transparent communication among members.

8. Decision-making process: Establish a decision-making process that ensures all members have a voice and their perspectives are considered. This may involve consensus-building, voting, or utilizing the expertise of specific individuals for certain decisions. Encourage constructive discussions and find ways to reconcile differing viewpoints.

9. Regular evaluation and adjustment: Continuously evaluate the progress and effectiveness of the task force, work group, or team. Regularly assess the outcomes of the crisis management efforts and identify areas for improvement or adjustment. Incorporate feedback from stakeholders and adapt the strategies as needed.

10. Documentation and reporting: Maintain accurate and up-to-date documentation of the activities, decisions, and outcomes of the task force, work group, or team. This includes keeping records of meetings, progress reports, and any relevant data or evidence. Provide regular reports to stakeholders and communicate the achievements and challenges encountered.

Remember, flexibility and adaptability are crucial in the post-revolution crisis management context. Regularly review the composition, structure, and strategies of the task force, work group, or team to ensure they remain aligned with the changing needs and dynamics of the crisis.

Collaborating with international and humanitarian agencies in post-revolution healthcare system crises involves a series of processes and procedures. Here are some key steps to consider:

1. Needs assessment: Conduct a thorough assessment of the healthcare system, identifying areas of immediate concern and specific needs. This assessment should help determine the type and level of support required from international and humanitarian agencies.

2. Identify potential partners: Research and identify international and humanitarian agencies that have experience in post-conflict healthcare crises and align with the goals and needs of your country. Consider organizations such as the World Health Organization (WHO), Médecins Sans Frontières (MSF), International Committee of the Red Cross (ICRC), or relevant United Nations agencies.

3. Contact and establish communication: Reach out to the identified agencies through official channels, such as their headquarters or regional offices. Initiate communication by explaining the healthcare crisis, the specific needs, and the desire to collaborate. Provide relevant background information and outline the potential areas of partnership.

4. Memorandum of Understanding (MoU): Once there is mutual interest in collaboration, establish a formal agreement through a Memorandum of Understanding (MoU). This document should outline the objectives, roles, responsibilities, and activities to be undertaken by both parties. It should also include provisions related to confidentiality, financial arrangements, reporting mechanisms, and duration of collaboration.

5. Resource mobilization: Collaborate with international and humanitarian agencies to secure the necessary resources, including funding, medical supplies, equipment, and technical expertise. Provide them with accurate information on the specific needs and prioritize areas where support is required.

6. Coordination mechanism: Establish a coordination mechanism involving local authorities, relevant government agencies, and international/humanitarian partners. This mechanism should facilitate regular communication, information sharing, and joint decision-making. It should also address any potential challenges or conflicts that may arise during the collaboration.

7. Capacity-building and training: Work with international and humanitarian agencies to develop capacity-building programs for local healthcare professionals and institutions. This may involve training programs, workshops, and knowledge transfer initiatives to enhance the skills and capacities of the local healthcare workforce.

8. Monitoring and evaluation: Develop a system for monitoring and evaluating the progress and impact of the collaborated activities. Regularly assess the effectiveness of the interventions, identify any gaps or challenges, and make adjustments as needed.

9. Reporting and accountability: Establish reporting mechanisms to provide regular updates to the international and humanitarian agencies on the progress, challenges, and outcomes of the collaboration. Ensure transparency and accountability in the use of resources and adherence to agreed-upon activities.

10. Long-term partnerships: Foster long-term partnerships with international and humanitarian agencies to support the sustainable development of the healthcare system. Explore opportunities for continued collaboration beyond the immediate crisis response, such as capacity-building initiatives, research collaborations, or policy development support.

Remember, the specific processes and procedures may vary depending on the context, organizations involved, and the nature of the healthcare crisis. It is essential to maintain open and regular communication with the international and humanitarian agencies throughout the collaboration to ensure effective coordination and maximize support for the post-revolution healthcare system crisis.

The role of army and military forces in healthcare crisis management in both urban and rural areas can be significant. Here are some key roles they can play:

1. Emergency response and disaster management: The army and military forces have the training, resources, and logistical capabilities to respond quickly to healthcare crises, such as natural disasters, pandemics, or other emergencies. They can provide immediate assistance in setting up field hospitals, triage centers, and temporary medical facilities in both urban and rural areas.

2. Infrastructure support: The army can assist in rebuilding or repairing damaged healthcare infrastructure, such as hospitals, clinics, and medical facilities, in post-crisis situations. They can provide manpower, equipment, and expertise to expedite the restoration of healthcare services.

3. Transportation and logistics: Military forces have well-established transportation and logistics capabilities. They can assist in the transportation of medical personnel, equipment, supplies, and patients, especially in remote or hard-to-reach rural areas. This is particularly crucial during healthcare crises when the regular transportation system may be disrupted.

4. Security and protection: During healthcare crises, maintaining law and order is essential to ensure the safety of healthcare professionals, patients, and medical facilities. The army and military forces can provide security and protection to healthcare workers, medical facilities, and supply routes, particularly in conflict-affected areas.

5. Humanitarian aid and outreach: Military forces often have access to resources and capabilities to provide humanitarian aid and outreach in healthcare crises. They can distribute essential supplies, provide medical assistance, and support vaccination campaigns in both urban and rural areas, especially when there are limited healthcare resources available.

6. Training and capacity building: The army and military forces can contribute to training healthcare personnel in disaster response, emergency medical care, and crisis management. They can share their expertise and experiences with healthcare professionals, community health workers, and volunteers to enhance their readiness and capabilities during future healthcare crises.

7. Coordination and collaboration: The army can play a crucial role in coordinating and collaborating with other stakeholders, including government agencies, non-governmental organizations (NGOs), and international partners. They can establish joint command centers, facilitate information sharing, and ensure effective coordination among various actors involved in healthcare crisis management.

However, it is important to note that the involvement of the army and military forces in healthcare crisis management should be governed by clear guidelines and principles. They should work in close collaboration with healthcare authorities and abide by medical ethics to ensure that healthcare interventions are provided in a manner that prioritizes the well-being and dignity of affected populations.

Post-revolution health system crisis management in rural areas requires a comprehensive approach to address the unique challenges faced by these communities. Here are some key steps to effectively manage the crisis:

1. Assess the situation: Conduct a thorough assessment of the health system in rural areas post-revolution. Identify the specific challenges, such as damaged infrastructure, limited access to healthcare services, shortage of healthcare professionals, and disrupted supply chains for medications and medical supplies.

2. Strengthen primary healthcare services: Focus on strengthening primary healthcare services, which play a crucial role in rural areas. This includes:

- Recruiting and training healthcare professionals: Recruit and train doctors, nurses, and community health workers to provide essential healthcare services in rural areas. Offer incentives to attract healthcare professionals to work in these underserved areas.

- Enhancing healthcare infrastructure: Repair or rebuild damaged healthcare facilities. Establish new primary healthcare centers or clinics in areas lacking access to healthcare. Ensure these facilities have the necessary equipment, supplies, and basic amenities.

- Promoting preventive care: Emphasize health promotion and disease prevention through education campaigns, vaccinations, and screenings. Encourage and educate the community on adopting healthy behaviors and practices.

3. Mobile clinics and outreach services: Deploy mobile clinics and outreach teams to reach remote and underserved areas in rural regions. These teams can provide primary healthcare services, health education, and screenings. Collaborate with local community leaders and organizations to ensure effective outreach and coordination.

4. Telemedicine and technology: Utilize telemedicine and technology to bridge the gap in healthcare access in rural areas. This includes:

- Establishing telemedicine networks: Develop telemedicine networks to connect rural healthcare providers with specialists in urban areas. This allows for remote consultations, diagnosis, and treatment.

- Mobile health applications: Promote the use of mobile health applications that provide health information, remote monitoring, and appointment scheduling. Ensure access to reliable internet connectivity in rural areas to facilitate the use of such technologies.

5. Strengthen supply chains: Address disruptions in the supply chains for medications and medical supplies by:

- Establishing central distribution centers: Set up central distribution centers in strategic locations to ensure efficient and timely delivery of medications and medical supplies to rural areas.

- Collaboration with NGOs and international organizations: Collaborate with NGOs and international organizations specializing in healthcare supply chain management to ensure a steady flow of essential medical resources to rural areas.

6. Community engagement and empowerment: Engage and empower local communities to take an active role in their healthcare:

- Community health workers: Train and deploy community health workers who can provide basic healthcare services, and health education, and act as a link between the community and healthcare providers.

- Community health committees: Establish community health committees comprising local representatives, healthcare professionals, and community members to identify and address healthcare needs, ensure accountability, and advocate for necessary resources.

7. Monitoring and evaluation: Regularly monitor and evaluate the effectiveness of the implemented strategies in rural areas. Assess the impact, identify gaps, and make necessary adjustments to improve the healthcare services and crisis management efforts.

Overall, a multi-faceted approach that combines strengthening primary healthcare, utilizing mobile clinics and technology, ensuring a robust supply chain, and empowering local communities is essential for effective post-revolution health system crisis management in rural areas.

Managing and distributing food and medications in a post-revolution crisis requires careful planning, coordination, and collaboration among various stakeholders. Here are some key considerations for effective food and medication management:

1. Assess needs and prioritize: Conduct a comprehensive assessment to understand the immediate and long-term needs of the population regarding food and medications.

Prioritize vulnerable groups such as children, the elderly, pregnant women, and individuals with chronic illnesses.

2. Establish supply chains: Identify and establish reliable supply chains for food and medications. This may involve collaborating with local and international suppliers, NGOs, and humanitarian organizations. Ensure the supply chains are resilient and can withstand potential disruptions.

3. Centralize coordination: Establish a centralized coordination mechanism to oversee the management and distribution of food and medications. This can be done through a dedicated task force or committee that includes representatives from relevant government agencies, NGOs, healthcare providers, and community leaders.

4. Inventory management: Implement robust inventory management systems to track and monitor the availability of food and medications. This includes regular stock assessments, forecasting, and replenishment processes to ensure adequate supplies are maintained. Utilize technology, such as barcode scanning or digital tracking systems, to improve accuracy and efficiency.

5. Distribution planning: Develop a distribution plan that outlines the logistics, routes, and timelines for delivering food and medications to the affected areas. Consider the accessibility of the locations, transportation options, and security measures. Collaborate with local authorities and community leaders to ensure effective distribution.

6. Community engagement: Engage with the local communities to understand their specific needs, preferences, and cultural considerations related to food and medications. Involve community leaders and organizations in the distribution process to ensure transparency, accountability, and acceptance of the assistance provided.

7. Ensure quality and safety: Establish stringent quality control measures to ensure the safety and efficacy of food and medications. Adhere to national and international standards for food safety and pharmaceutical regulations. Regularly inspect and monitor the storage and distribution facilities to prevent spoilage, contamination, or expiration of products.

8. Information dissemination: Develop a comprehensive communication strategy to inform the affected population about the availability, distribution points, and proper usage of food and medications. Utilize various channels such as radio, television, social media, and community networks to reach a wide audience. Provide clear instructions and warnings regarding any potential risks or side effects.

9. Monitoring and evaluation: Implement a robust monitoring and evaluation system to assess the effectiveness and impact of the food and medication management and distribution efforts. Regularly collect feedback from the beneficiaries and stakeholders to identify any gaps or areas for improvement. Use this information to adapt and refine the strategies.

10. Collaborate with international organizations: Seek support and collaboration from international organizations, such as the World Food Program (WFP) and the World Health Organization (WHO). They can provide technical expertise, funding, and coordination support to enhance food and medication management efforts.

Remember, it is essential to prioritize the well-being and dignity of the affected population throughout the food and medication management process. Ensure equitable distribution, respect cultural preferences, and maintain transparency to build trust and foster resilience in the post-revolution crisis context!

In post-revolution crises, when healthcare infrastructure may be damaged or inaccessible, temporary medical homes, mobile clinics, and tent clinics can play a crucial role in providing essential healthcare services to both urban and rural areas. Here's how they can be effectively implemented:

1. Temporary Medical Homes:

- Identify suitable locations: Select appropriate buildings or facilities, such as schools, community centers, or vacant buildings, to set up temporary medical homes. Consider their proximity to the affected population and availability of basic amenities like water and electricity.

- Equip and staff the facilities: Equip the temporary medical homes with necessary medical equipment, supplies, and basic furniture. Recruit healthcare professionals, including doctors, nurses, and support staff, to provide healthcare services.

- Offer comprehensive care: Provide primary healthcare services, including general consultations, vaccinations, basic laboratory tests, and essential medications. Collaborate with local health authorities and NGOs to ensure the availability of specialized care and referrals for more complex cases.

- Establish infection control measures: Implement strict infection control protocols, including hand hygiene, waste management, and patient triage, to prevent the spread of diseases within the temporary medical homes.

2. Mobile Clinics:

- Assess target areas: Identify areas with limited access to healthcare services, both in urban and rural settings. Assess the population density, health needs, and transportation logistics to determine the most suitable locations for mobile clinics.

- Retrofit vehicles: Convert vans or buses into mobile clinics by equipping them with basic medical equipment, examination tables, and storage for medications and supplies. Ensure the vehicles comply with safety and hygiene standards.

- Schedule regular visits: Develop a schedule for mobile clinic visits to different locations, considering the specific needs and availability of the target population. Coordinate with local community leaders and organizations to spread awareness and facilitate patient appointments.

- Provide preventive and curative services: Offer a range of healthcare services, including general check-ups, vaccinations, health education, and treatment for common illnesses. Maintain a stock of essential medications and supplies to address immediate healthcare needs.

- Collaborate with local resources: Partner with local healthcare providers, community health workers, and volunteers to enhance the reach and effectiveness of mobile clinics. This collaboration can help identify priority areas, establish trust, and provide continuity of care beyond the mobile clinic visits.

3. Tent Clinics:

- Identify suitable locations: In rural areas or areas with limited infrastructure, tent clinics can be set up to provide basic healthcare services. Identify open spaces or community centers where tents can be installed.

- Ensure basic facilities: Set up tents with separate areas for patient consultations, waiting areas, and storage of medical supplies. Ensure access to clean water, sanitation facilities, and electricity where possible.

- Organize outreach teams: Deploy healthcare professionals, including doctors, nurses, and support staff, to the tent clinics. Organize outreach teams to visit the surrounding areas and inform the community about the services available.

- Offer primary care services: Provide primary healthcare services, including consultations, basic diagnostics, wound care, and medication distribution. Collaborate with local health authorities to ensure access to specialized care and referrals as needed.

- Address community-specific needs: Adapt services to meet the specific needs of the community, such as providing maternal and child healthcare, mental health support, or chronic disease management. Engage with community leaders and representatives to understand and address their healthcare priorities.

In all these approaches, it is essential to establish strong coordination with local health authorities, NGOs, and community leaders to ensure the effective management and sustainability of temporary medical homes, mobile clinics, and tent clinics. Regular monitoring and evaluation should be conducted to assess the impact and address any challenges that arise during the post-revolution crisis.

In a post-revolution scenario in a failed state, re-installing the previous healthcare worker's conditions and requirements can be a complex and challenging task. Here are some considerations for this process:

1. Assess the existing healthcare workforce: Evaluate the current state of the healthcare workforce, including the number of available healthcare workers, their qualifications, and

their willingness to return to work. This assessment will help determine the capacity and readiness of the healthcare system.

2. Address grievances and incentives: Engage with healthcare workers to understand their concerns and grievances. Address any issues related to salaries, working conditions, security, and professional development opportunities. Providing incentives, such as improved remuneration packages and career advancement prospects, can help attract and retain qualified healthcare workers.

3. Re-establish regulatory bodies: Restore or establish regulatory bodies responsible for setting standards, licensing, and accreditation of healthcare professionals. These bodies should ensure that healthcare workers meet the required qualifications and adhere to ethical and professional guidelines.

4. Training and capacity building: Develop comprehensive training programs to enhance the skills and knowledge of healthcare workers. This can include refresher courses, continuing education programs, and specialized training in areas that are particularly relevant to the post-revolution context, such as trauma care or mental health support.

5. Recruitment and deployment: Develop transparent and fair recruitment processes to attract qualified healthcare workers. Consider establishing recruitment committees or boards that include representatives from healthcare professional associations, civil society organizations, and relevant government bodies. Ensure that the recruitment process is merit-based and free from political interference.

6. Strengthen healthcare infrastructure: Rebuilding and strengthening healthcare infrastructure, including hospitals, clinics, and medical facilities, is crucial for providing quality healthcare services. Invest in infrastructure development, equipment procurement, and maintenance to create an enabling environment for healthcare workers to deliver effective care.

7. Collaborate with international partners: Seek support and collaboration from international organizations, NGOs, and donor agencies to aid in the re-establishment of the healthcare system. International partners can provide technical expertise, financial resources, and assistance in capacity-building efforts.

8. Monitor and evaluate progress: Establish monitoring and evaluation mechanisms to assess the effectiveness of the re-installed healthcare worker conditions and requirements. Monitor workforce distribution, patient outcomes, and healthcare worker satisfaction to identify areas for improvement and ensure accountability.

It is important to note that re-installing the previous healthcare worker's conditions and requirements may not be sufficient in a post-revolution scenario. It is essential to address the underlying systemic issues that led to the failure of the state and the healthcare system. Comprehensive reforms, including governance, policy development, and financial sustainability, are crucial for long-term success.

In a post-revolution scenario, the reinstatement of healthcare workers who were illegitimately fired or forced into retirement is an important step toward rectifying past injustices. Here are some considerations for their reinstatement:

1. Conduct a thorough review: Initiate a comprehensive review of the circumstances surrounding the illegitimate firing or forced retirement of healthcare workers. This review should involve gathering evidence, interviewing relevant parties, and consulting legal experts, if necessary. Identify cases where clear violations of labor laws or human rights occurred.

2. Ensure due process: In cases where illegitimate actions are identified, ensure that due process is followed. This may involve re-opening investigations, providing opportunities for affected healthcare workers to present their cases, and addressing any procedural or legal shortcomings that occurred during the original termination or retirement process.

3. Provide compensation and restitution: If it is determined that healthcare workers were unjustly fired or forced into retirement, provide appropriate compensation and restitution for the damages they incurred. This could include back pay, reinstatement with seniority and benefits restored, and any other necessary measures to restore their professional standing.

4. Support reintegration and professional development: Offer support and resources to facilitate the reintegration and professional development of the reinstated healthcare workers. This may involve providing training programs, mentorship opportunities, or access to continuing education to help them update their skills and adapt to any changes in the healthcare landscape.

5. Foster a supportive work environment: Create a work environment that is supportive and inclusive for the reinstated healthcare workers. Encourage open communication, collaboration, and respect among all healthcare professionals. Address any potential conflicts or tensions that may arise from the reintegration process and promote a culture of teamwork and professional growth.

6. Monitor workplace dynamics: Implement mechanisms to monitor workplace dynamics and ensure that the reinstated healthcare workers are treated fairly and without prejudice. This can involve regular evaluations, feedback mechanisms, and addressing any discriminatory practices or behavior that may hinder their reintegration.

7. Promote transparency and accountability: Maintain transparency throughout the process of reinstating healthcare workers. Communicate the reasons for their reinstatement to the public, ensuring that they understand the rationale behind rectifying past injustices. Hold accountable those responsible for the illegitimate actions, if applicable, to prevent future occurrences.

8. Learn from past mistakes: Use the experiences and lessons learned from the illegitimate firing or forced retirement cases to improve healthcare policies, procedures, and oversight

mechanisms. Implement safeguards to prevent similar injustices from happening in the future and ensure that all healthcare workers are treated fairly and equitably.

Reinstating healthcare workers who were illegitimately fired or forced into retirement is a crucial step in restoring trust, promoting justice, and building a more inclusive and effective healthcare system in the post-revolution era. It requires a commitment to fairness, transparency, and accountability, and should be guided by the overarching goal of providing quality healthcare to all individuals.

In a post-revolution scenario, the reinstatement of healthcare workers who were illegitimately fired or forced into retirement is an important step toward rectifying past injustices. Here are some considerations for their reinstatement:

1. Conduct a thorough review: Initiate a comprehensive review of the circumstances surrounding the illegitimate firing or forced retirement of healthcare workers. This review should involve gathering evidence, interviewing relevant parties, and consulting legal experts, if necessary. Identify cases where clear violations of labor laws or human rights occurred.

2. Ensure due process: In cases where illegitimate actions are identified, ensure that due process is followed. This may involve re-opening investigations, providing opportunities for affected healthcare workers to present their cases, and addressing any procedural or legal shortcomings that occurred during the original termination or retirement process.

3. Provide compensation and restitution: If it is determined that healthcare workers were unjustly fired or forced into retirement, provide appropriate compensation and restitution for the damages they incurred. This could include back pay, reinstatement with seniority and benefits restored, and any other necessary measures to restore their professional standing.

4. Support reintegration and professional development: Offer support and resources to facilitate the reintegration and professional development of the reinstated healthcare workers. This may involve providing training programs, mentorship opportunities, or access to continuing education to help them update their skills and adapt to any changes in the healthcare landscape.

5. Foster a supportive work environment: Create a work environment that is supportive and inclusive for the reinstated healthcare workers. Encourage open communication, collaboration, and respect among all healthcare professionals. Address any potential conflicts or tensions that may arise from the reintegration process and promote a culture of teamwork and professional growth.

6. Monitor workplace dynamics: Implement mechanisms to monitor workplace dynamics and ensure that the reinstated healthcare workers are treated fairly and without prejudice. This can involve regular evaluations, feedback mechanisms, and addressing any discriminatory practices or behavior that may hinder their reintegration.

7. Promote transparency and accountability: Maintain transparency throughout the process of reinstating healthcare workers. Communicate the reasons for their reinstatement to the public, ensuring that they understand the rationale behind rectifying past injustices. Hold accountable those responsible for the illegitimate actions, if applicable, to prevent future occurrences.

8. Learn from past mistakes: Use the experiences and lessons learned from the illegitimate firing or forced retirement cases to improve healthcare policies, procedures, and oversight mechanisms. Implement safeguards to prevent similar injustices from happening in the future and ensure that all healthcare workers are treated fairly and equitably.

Reinstating healthcare workers who were illegitimately fired or forced into retirement is a crucial step in restoring trust, promoting justice, and building a more inclusive and effective healthcare system in the post-revolution era. It requires a commitment to fairness, transparency, and accountability, and should be guided by the overarching goal of providing quality healthcare to all individuals.

Islamic Republic of Iran chemical warfare

Introduction

Chemical warfare refers to the use of toxic chemicals as weapons to cause harm, incapacitate, or kill humans, animals, or plants. It is a form of warfare that has been prohibited by various international treaties and conventions due to the severe and indiscriminate nature of its effects. Despite these bans, chemical weapons have been used in conflicts throughout history, causing immense suffering and devastation.

Chemical weapons can be classified into several categories, including nerve agents, blister agents, choking agents, blood agents, and riot control agents. Nerve agents, such as sarin and VX, disrupt the normal functioning of the nervous system, leading to paralysis and, in high doses, respiratory failure and death. Blister agents, like mustard gas, cause severe blistering of the skin, eyes, and respiratory tract. Choking agents, such as chlorine and phosgene, damage lung tissue, leading to suffocation. Blood agents, like cyanide compounds, interfere with the body's ability to utilize oxygen, causing asphyxiation. Riot control agents, such as tear gas, are less lethal and primarily used for temporary incapacitation or dispersing crowds.

The use of chemical weapons is considered a violation of international law and various treaties. The most notable treaty addressing chemical warfare is the Chemical Weapons Convention (CWC), which prohibits the development, production, stockpiling, and use of chemical weapons. The CWC, which entered into force in 1997, has been ratified by almost all nations, making it one of the most comprehensive disarmament treaties.

The effects of chemical warfare can be long-lasting and devastating. Exposure to chemical agents can cause immediate symptoms such as respiratory distress, eye irritation, skin burns, and neurological impairment. Chronic exposure may lead to long-term health complications, including respiratory problems, cancer, and psychological trauma.

Efforts to prevent the use of chemical weapons include international inspections and monitoring, destruction of stockpiles, and promoting awareness and adherence to the Chemical Weapons Convention. Organizations like the Organization for the Prohibition of Chemical Weapons (OPCW) play a crucial role in enforcing the treaty and conducting investigations into alleged chemical weapons use.

In conclusion, chemical warfare is a barbaric and inhumane method of warfare that causes immense suffering and long-term consequences. The international community continues to work towards eliminating chemical weapons and enforcing the treaties and conventions designed to protect humanity from their use.

Islamic Republic of Iran Possible Chemical Weapon Arsenals:

It's important to note that the use of chemical weapons is strictly prohibited by international law. information about the Islamic Republic's chemical weapons and list of the gases in their arsenals are scarce and mostly unconfirmed or denied by the Iranian government. However, there are some reports regarding the Islamic Republic providing and using chemical weapons in Syria and against the Kurdish population. Recent chemical gas usage in girl's elementary, middle, and high school is another piece of evidence that raises the possibility of the usage of chemical weapons by the Iranian government against people and protestors. This possibility is highly concerning and should be condemned and reported.

Possible Islamic Republic exciting Chemical Arsenals:

Some common types of chemical gases that have been historically used as weapons include:

1. Nerve Agents: Examples of nerve agents include Sarin, VX, and Tabun. These highly toxic substances interfere with the functioning of the nervous system, causing paralysis and, in severe cases, leading to respiratory failure.
2. Blister Agents: Mustard gas (Sulfur Mustard) and Lewisite are examples of blister agents. These gases cause severe burns, blistering, and tissue damage on contact with the skin or eyes.
3. Choking Agents: Chlorine and Phosgene are examples of choking agents. These gases cause severe irritation to the respiratory system, leading to symptoms such as coughing, difficulty breathing, and potentially fatal lung damage.
4. Blood Agents: Hydrogen Cyanide and Cyanogen Chloride are examples of blood agents. These gases interfere with the body's ability to utilize oxygen, leading to asphyxiation.

Nitrogen Gas Allegedly Used in Girl's School:

Exposure to nitrogen gas can be dangerous, especially in enclosed spaces where it can displace oxygen. The treatment for nitrogen gas exposure primarily focuses on ensuring adequate oxygen supply and addressing any complications that may arise. Here are some general guidelines for treatment:

1. Move to fresh air: If you suspect nitrogen gas exposure, immediately move the affected person to an area with fresh air. Ensure proper ventilation to reduce the concentration of nitrogen gas.
2. Administer oxygen: If the person is having trouble breathing or shows signs of oxygen deprivation, administer supplemental oxygen if available. This can help restore adequate oxygen levels in the body.
3. Provide supportive care: Monitor the person's vital signs, including heart rate, blood pressure, and oxygen saturation levels. If any complications arise, such as respiratory

distress or cardiac abnormalities, seek immediate medical attention.

4. Seek medical evaluation: Even if the initial symptoms improve, it is essential to seek medical evaluation to assess the extent of exposure and any potential complications that may develop later.
5. It is important to note that nitrogen gas exposure is often a result of oxygen displacement, leading to oxygen deprivation or asphyxiation. Thus, the primary focus is on ensuring adequate oxygen supply and promptly seeking medical evaluation for further assessment and care.

Emergency Treatment and Medical Attention:

The treatment for exposure to chemical gases depends on the specific gas involved. It is crucial to seek immediate medical attention if you or someone else has been exposed to a chemical gas. Here are some general guidelines for treatment:

1. Nerve Agents (e.g., Sarin, VX, Tabun):

- Move to fresh air immediately.

- Remove contaminated clothing and rinse the body with water.

- Atropine and pralidoxime chloride are specific antidotes used to counter the effects of nerve agents. Medical professionals administer these antidotes.

2. Blister Agents (e.g., Mustard Gas, Lewisite):

- Move to fresh air and remove contaminated clothing.

- Rinse the affected area with copious amounts of water.

- Apply a sterile dressing to protect the blisters and prevent infection.

- Seek medical treatment for further evaluation and care.

3. Choking Agents (e.g., Chlorine, Phosgene):

- Move to fresh air immediately.

- If breathing is difficult, administer oxygen if available.

- Seek immediate medical attention.

4. Blood Agents (e.g., Hydrogen Cyanide, Cyanogen Chloride):

- Move to fresh air immediately.

- Administer oxygen if available.

- Seek immediate medical attention.

It is important to note that these are general guidelines, and the specific treatment for chemical gas exposure should be determined by medical professionals based on the individual circumstances and the gas involved. Following exposure, it is crucial to decontaminate the affected individuals and the environment appropriately.

Islamic Republic of Iran
Medical Education and Professionalism Disparities, Failures, and Solutions

The IR constitution defines the country as an Islamic republic and specifies Twelve Ja'afari.

Shai Islam is the official state religion.

It states all laws and regulations must be based on Islamic Criteria and an official interpretation of Sharia.

The constitution states citizens shall enjoy human, political, economic, and other rights in conformity with Islamic Criteria.

The penal code provides for hudud punishments including amputation, flogging, and stoning (Iran 2022 International Religious Freedom Report).

Sharia law refers to the legal system based on the principles of Islamic religious teachings, primarily derived from the Quran and the Hadith (sayings and actions of Prophet Muhammad). It governs various aspects of life, including personal behavior, family matters, business transactions, and criminal justice. It serves as a moral and ethical guide for Muslims and aims to promote justice, equality, and the well-being of society.

Sharia law encompasses a wide range of topics, such as marriage, divorce, inheritance, contracts, and criminal offenses. It places great emphasis on mutual respect, fairness, and compassion. It seeks to protect individual rights and promote social welfare, encouraging charitable acts and helping those in need.

Under Sharia law in Iran, women have certain rights and responsibilities, but it's important to note that interpretations and implementations can vary. Here's a general overview:

1. Life: Women in Iran have the right to life and personal safety, just like men. However, certain behaviors or choices that are considered against Islamic principles may face stricter punishments or societal pressures.
2. Education: Women have access to education in Iran, and there are no legal restrictions on their right to education. However, societal factors and cultural norms can sometimes limit educational opportunities for women, particularly in more conservative areas.
3. Marriage: Under Sharia law, women have the right to consent to marriage and cannot be forced into marriage against their will. However, certain legal and cultural practices can undermine this right in some cases. Polygamy is allowed in Iran, but a man must obtain permission from a court and prove his ability to treat all wives

equally.

4. Inheritance: Sharia law prescribes specific rules for inheritance. In Iran, women generally have the right to inherit property, but the share they receive can be different from that of men. For example, a daughter may receive half the share of a son. However, it's worth noting that recent legal reforms in Iran have aimed to address gender disparities in inheritance rights.
5. It's important to remember that these are general points, and the actual lived experiences of Iranian women can vary depending on various factors such as regional customs, socio-economic status, and personal circumstances.

Medical Education and Healthcare System Delivery:

The current quota system in the Islamic Republic of Iran aims to promote equal opportunities for underrepresented groups in medical school admission. The quota system intends a certain number of seats for specific categories of applicants, including students from rural areas, ethnic minorities, and individuals with disabilities which in reality is ignored and overlooked. The purpose of this system is to address presumed historical inequalities and increase access to higher education for marginalized populations.

The specific details of the quota system can vary from year to year, but generally, it involves allocating a certain percentage of seats in medical schools to applicants from these underrepresented groups. For example, a certain percentage of seats may be reserved for students from rural areas, regardless of their performance in the entrance exams, merit, and educational aptitude. However, the Islamic Republic ignores its mandated policies and instead, a certain number of seats are reserved for individuals who have demonstrated a commitment to the Islamic faith and have a strong religious background. Additionally, there may be a quota for the children of war martyrs who are given preferential treatment in the admission process.

These policies aim to promote the values and principles of the Islamic Republic of Iran and ensure that individuals with strong religious beliefs have opportunities to pursue professional education regardless of their eligibility, merit academic aptitude, and passing scores in entrance exams.

As a rule, the quota system is intended to provide opportunities to individuals who may face additional barriers to accessing quality education or achieving high scores in the highly competitive entrance exams. By reserving a certain number of seats for these groups, the system in a free and democratic society aims to create a more diverse and inclusive medical student body.

However, the implementation and specific details of the quota system have been the subject of debate and criticism in Iran. Some argue that the system may compromise merit-based admission and result in a lower standard of education in medical schools. Critics also express concerns that the system may be susceptible to abuse or manipulation, with applicants falsely claiming eligibility for quota seats.

It is important to note that the quota system is just one aspect of the medical school admission process in many countries. Other criteria, such as performance in specific and national exams and academic achievements, also play a significant role in determining admission. The quota system is meant to supplement these criteria and provide opportunities for underrepresented groups, but it does not solely determine admission outcomes Unfortunately none of the above criteria other than Islamic organization affiliation are observed in the Islamic Republic of Iran.

In Iran, like in many countries, disparities in medical school admission exist and can be attributed to various factors. Some of the main disparities in medical school admission in Iran include:

1. Regional Disparities: There is a significant regional imbalance in medical school admission in Iran. Students from wealthier or more developed regions tend to have better access to quality education and resources, which can give them an advantage in the highly competitive medical school entrance exams. As a result, students from less privileged regions may face additional barriers to gaining admission to medical schools.
2. Socioeconomic Disparities: Socioeconomic factors play a significant role in medical school admission disparities. Students from wealthier backgrounds often have access to better preparatory resources, such as private tutoring or specialized coaching classes, which can enhance their performance in entrance exams. On the other hand, students from lower-income families may face financial constraints and lack the resources necessary to compete on an equal footing.
3. Gender Disparities: Gender disparities can also be observed in medical school admission in Iran. While women make up a significant proportion of medical school applicants, there is a notable gender gap in terms of acceptance rates. This is due to various societal and cultural factors that may discourage or limit women's access to higher education, including medical schools.
4. Educational Disparities: Disparities in the quality of pre-university education can significantly impact medical school admission outcomes. Students from schools with limited resources, outdated curricula, and inadequate teaching staff may face challenges in acquiring the necessary knowledge and skills to perform well in entrance exams. This can disproportionately affect students from marginalized communities.
5. Merit vs. Quota System: The existence of quota systems in medical school admission can contribute to disparities. To promote equal opportunities for underrepresented groups, including students from rural areas or ethnic minorities, a certain number of seats may be reserved. While this aims to address inequalities, it can also create a

perception that some students are admitted based on factors other than merit, leading to concerns about fairness and competition.

Addressing these disparities requires a multi-faceted approach:

1. Equal Access to Quality Education: Improve the quality of pre-university education in underserved regions by investing in infrastructure, resources, and qualified teachers. This will help ensure that students from all regions have an equal opportunity to compete for medical school admission.
2. Targeted Support Programs: Implement targeted support programs, such as scholarship initiatives and mentoring programs, to assist students from disadvantaged backgrounds. These programs can provide financial support, guidance, and resources to help students overcome barriers and compete on an equal footing.
3. Awareness and Outreach: Increase awareness about medical school admission requirements, entrance exams, and available support programs among potential applicants. This can be achieved through targeted outreach campaigns, workshops, and information sessions in schools and communities.
4. Reforming Admission Processes: Continuously review and reform the medical school admission processes to ensure they are fair, transparent, and merit-based. This may involve reducing or eliminating quota systems while still considering the need to address historical inequalities and promote diversity.
5. Gender Equality Promotion: Encourage and support women's participation in higher education, including medical schools, through targeted initiatives, scholarships, and awareness campaigns. Address cultural and societal barriers that discourage women from pursuing medical careers.
6. Collaboration and Research: Foster collaboration between educational institutions, government bodies, and relevant stakeholders to research admission disparities and develop evidence-based strategies for addressing them effectively.

By addressing these disparities in medical school admission, Iran can create a more equitable and inclusive healthcare system, ensuring that talented and deserving individuals from all backgrounds have the opportunity to pursue careers in medicine and contribute to the betterment of society

The current quota system in general and in medical education in particular, not only has negatively impacted medical and higher medical education but also has resulted in lower educational and training quality and standard and quality of care delivery.

The Islamic cultural revolution and applied Islamic criteria and quotas to the selection process and retaining academic staff and teachers have dramatically and negatively impacted the quality of higher medical education, specialty training, and practice of medicine in the country.

Many academic staff and leaders have been forced to retire or have been expunged.

Many of those medical school graduates also received preferential quota placement and entered specialty training with out taking entrance exam, leaving those with higher scores behind the closed doors.

The followings are the examples of quota assigned admission to specialty training for academic year 2022-2023:

1-Radiology and Nuclear Medicine > 50%

2- Orthopedic Surgery > 69%

3- Cardiovascular Disease > 62%

This trend applies to all trainings in country.

Rebuilding and remedial needs:

This process is multifaceted and requires large and qualified personnel and task force. In all three sections, medical school, specialty and residency and practicing physicians and healthcare force.

1. Program Assessment and Identification:

- Conduct a thorough assessment of the current situation, including the admission process, curriculum, and competency levels of the affected physicians.

- Identify the specific religious or political connections that influenced their admission and evaluate the impact on their medical knowledge and skills.

- Collaborate with local healthcare authorities, educational institutions, and professional associations to develop a targeted retraining program.

2. Preparatory Courses:

- Offer preparatory courses to bridge knowledge gaps in basic medical sciences, such as anatomy, physiology, biochemistry, and pharmacology.

- Provide comprehensive lectures, interactive sessions, and practical demonstrations to ensure a strong foundation in essential medical concepts.

- Utilize modern teaching methodologies, including case-based learning and problem-solving exercises, to promote critical thinking and clinical reasoning.

3. Clinical Training and Skill Development:

- Arrange clinical rotations and internships in reputable healthcare institutions to provide hands-on experience under the guidance of experienced physicians.

- Focus on enhancing clinical skills, including history taking, physical examination, diagnostic reasoning, and evidence-based treatment planning.

- Provide opportunities for physicians to observe and participate in various medical procedures, surgeries, and specialized clinics relevant to their chosen specialties.

4. Specialty-Specific Education:

- Tailor the retraining program to each physician's desired specialty, such as internal medicine, surgery, pediatrics, or obstetrics and gynecology.

- Offer specialty-specific lectures, workshops, and case discussions to deepen their understanding and practical skills in their chosen field.

- Engage specialists from various disciplines to provide comprehensive and up-to-date knowledge, fostering a multidisciplinary approach.

5. Professional Ethics and Communication Skills:

- Conduct workshops and seminars on medical ethics, professionalism, and effective communication skills.

- Emphasize the importance of patient-centered care, cultural sensitivity, and respect for diverse religious and political beliefs.

- Engage physicians in role-playing exercises, simulated patient interactions, and discussions on challenging ethical dilemmas to enhance their decision-making skills.

6. Continuous Medical Education:

- Establish a framework for continuous medical education to ensure physicians stay updated with the latest medical advancements and evidence-based practices.

- Provide access to online resources, medical journals, conferences, and workshops to support ongoing learning and professional growth.

- Encourage physicians to participate in research activities, present scientific papers, and contribute to medical literature to foster intellectual development.

7. Mentorship and Support:

- Assign experienced physicians as mentors to provide guidance, support, and career advice throughout the retraining program.

- Facilitate regular mentorship sessions to discuss challenges, set goals, and monitor progress, ensuring personalized support for each physician.

- Foster a supportive community by organizing networking events, peer-to-peer learning opportunities, and mentor-led discussions.

8. Program Evaluation and Monitoring:

- Establish an evaluation framework to assess the effectiveness of the retraining program and monitor the progress of participating physicians.

- Collect feedback from participants, mentors, and healthcare employers to identify strengths, weaknesses, and areas requiring improvement.

- Utilize evaluation results to refine the program, update curriculum content, adjust teaching methodologies, and address emerging needs.

9. Collaboration and Partnerships:

- Collaborate with local and international stakeholders, including healthcare institutions, professional associations, NGOs, and funding agencies.

- Seek partnerships with reputable medical schools or organizations to enhance program credibility and provide additional resources.

- Engage with policymakers and advocacy groups to address systemic issues and promote merit-based admission processes in medical education.

10. Sustainability and Long-Term Impact:

- Foster local ownership by involving local healthcare authorities, medical institutions, and professional associations in program planning and implementation.

- Develop a sustainability plan to ensure the program's continuity beyond the initial retraining phase, including strategies for financial support and resource management.

- Monitor the long-term impact of the program by tracking the professional success, career progression, and contributions of the retrained physicians to the healthcare sector.

By implementing this comprehensive retraining program, we aim to empower physicians who were admitted based on religious or political connections to acquire the necessary medical knowledge, skills, and ethical values. This program seeks to bridge the educational gaps and ensure that these physicians can provide high-quality, evidence-based healthcare, thereby improving the overall healthcare system in third-world countries.

Allied Health Professional Remedial and retraining:

This is a comprehensive program to retrain allied healthcare professionals in Iran during transition and freedom who were admitted to professional schools based on religious or political connections rather than merit or aptitude:

1.Program Assessment and Planning:

- Conduct a thorough assessment of the current situation, including the admission process, curriculum, and competency levels of the allied healthcare professionals.

- Identify the specific religious or political connections that affected their admission and evaluate the impact on their knowledge and skills.

- Collaborate with local healthcare authorities, educational institutions, and professional associations to develop a comprehensive retraining program.

2. Remedial Education and Skill Development:

- Offer foundational courses to bridge knowledge gaps in basic healthcare sciences, including anatomy, physiology, pharmacology, and medical terminology.

- Provide specialized training to enhance practical skills and competence in their respective allied healthcare fields, such as nursing, medical technology, or physiotherapy.

- Utilize a combination of classroom lectures, hands-on training, simulation exercises, and practical application to reinforce learning.

3. Professional Ethics and Values:

- Conduct workshops and discussions on professional ethics, emphasizing the importance of merit-based admission, equality, and patient-centered care.

- Facilitate sessions on cultural sensitivity, diversity, and respect for religious or political beliefs while ensuring unbiased and evidence-based healthcare practice.

- Encourage open dialogue and critical thinking to challenge preconceived notions and promote ethical decision-making in healthcare settings.

4. Clinical Experience and Practical Exposure:

- Arrange clinical rotations, internships, or apprenticeships in reputable healthcare facilities to provide hands-on experience under the guidance of experienced professionals.

- Encourage active participation in patient care, diagnostic procedures, treatment planning, and interprofessional collaboration to develop practical skills and confidence.

- Monitor and evaluate performance during clinical experiences to provide constructive feedback and identify areas for improvement.

5. Leadership and Management Skills:

- Offer training in leadership and management skills to equip allied healthcare professionals with the ability to lead teams, ensure quality care, and advocate for patient rights.

- Develop courses on healthcare administration, resource management, and effective communication to enhance their roles as future leaders in the healthcare sector.

- Provide opportunities for project management and quality improvement initiatives to foster innovation and enhance their ability to address healthcare challenges.

6. Continuous Professional Development:

- Establish a framework for ongoing professional development to ensure the retraining professionals stay updated with advancements in their fields.

- Provide access to relevant continuing education resources, online courses, conferences, and workshops to support lifelong learning.

- Encourage participation in research activities, publication opportunities, and knowledge-sharing platforms to foster professional growth and contribute to the healthcare community.

7. Mentorship and Support:

- Assign experienced allied healthcare professionals as mentors to provide guidance, support, and career advice throughout the retraining program.

- Facilitate regular mentorship sessions to discuss challenges, set goals, and monitor progress, ensuring personalized support for each retraining professional.

- Foster a supportive community by organizing networking events, peer-to-peer learning opportunities, and mentor-led discussions.

8. Program Evaluation and Monitoring:

- Establish an evaluation framework to monitor the effectiveness of the retraining program and assess the retraining professionals' progress.

- Collect feedback from participants, mentors, and healthcare employers to identify strengths, weaknesses, and areas requiring improvement.

- Use evaluation results to refine the program, update curriculum content, adjust teaching methodologies, and address emerging needs.

9. Collaboration and Partnerships:

- Collaborate with local and international stakeholders, including healthcare institutions, professional associations, NGOs, and funding agencies.

- Seek partnerships with reputable educational institutions or organizations to enhance program credibility and provide additional resources.

- Engage with policymakers and advocacy groups to address systemic issues and promote merit-based admission processes in allied healthcare education.

10. Sustainability and Long-Term Impact:

- Foster local ownership by involving local healthcare authorities, educational institutions, and professional associations in program planning and implementation.

- Develop a sustainability plan to ensure the program's continuity beyond the initial retraining phase, including strategies for financial support and resource management.

- Monitor the long-term impact of the program by tracking the professional success, career progression, and contributions of the retraining professionals to the healthcare sector.

Implementing this comprehensive retraining program requires strong collaboration among various stakeholders, meticulous planning, and ongoing evaluation. By addressing the educational gaps caused by religious or political connections, this program aims to empower allied healthcare professionals to deliver high-quality, patient-centered care based on merit and aptitude.

Pharmacy and related Industries:

Here is a comprehensive program to retrain pharmacists in Iran during transition and after people victory who were admitted to professional schools based on religious or political connections rather than merit or aptitude:

1. Program Orientation and Needs Assessment:

- Conduct an orientation session to explain the program's objectives, expectations, and benefits to the pharmacists.

- Administer a comprehensive needs assessment to identify their individual strengths, weaknesses, and areas requiring improvement.

- Gather data on their pharmacy education background, pharmaceutical knowledge, clinical skills, and personal goals.

2. Core Pharmaceutical Knowledge Enhancement:

- Provide intensive training in core pharmaceutical knowledge, including pharmacology, pharmaceutics, pharmacokinetics, and pharmacotherapy, to ensure a strong foundation.

- Offer specialized courses and workshops to update pharmacists on the latest drug information, evidence-based practice, and global health issues.

- Utilize interactive teaching methods, case studies, and practical exercises to enhance critical thinking and problem-solving skills.

3. Clinical Skills Development:

- Conduct hands-on training sessions to improve clinical skills, including medication dispensing, drug interactions screening, patient counseling, and medication therapy management.

- Provide simulated patient encounters and pharmacy simulations to practice and refine clinical skills in a controlled environment.

- Offer guidance on effective communication with patients, healthcare providers, and other members of the healthcare team to ensure patient-centered care.

4. Pharmaceutical Care and Patient Safety:

- Emphasize the importance of pharmaceutical care and patient safety in the practice of pharmacy.

- Provide training on medication reconciliation, adverse drug event reporting, medication error prevention, and quality assurance in pharmacy practice.

- Encourage pharmacists to develop patient monitoring plans, assess therapeutic outcomes, and collaborate with healthcare teams to optimize patient care.

5. Specialized Training and Continuing Education:

- Develop specialized training modules based on the pharmacists' areas of interest or the healthcare needs of their communities.

- Offer continuing pharmacy education (CPE) courses, conferences, and workshops to keep the pharmacists updated with the latest research, guidelines, and best practices.

- Collaborate with local and international pharmacy experts to deliver specialized training and share their expertise.

6. Ethical and Professional Development:

- Conduct sessions on pharmacy ethics, professional integrity, and patient confidentiality to reinforce the importance of ethical conduct in pharmacy practice.

- Promote evidence-based practice and encourage pharmacists to base their clinical decisions on scientific research and patient well-being.

- Facilitate discussions on the impact of religious or political influences on the pharmaceutical sector and emphasize the need for unbiased and patient-centered care.

7. Mentoring and Individual Support:

- Assign experienced pharmacists as mentors to provide one-on-one guidance, support, and career advice to the retraining pharmacists.

- Conduct regular mentorship sessions to address individual concerns, monitor progress, and provide feedback on clinical skills and professional development.

- Encourage retraining pharmacists to seek advice and share experiences with their mentors, promoting a supportive learning environment.

8. Practical Exposure and Internships:

- Collaborate with local healthcare institutions, community pharmacies, and pharmaceutical companies to provide practical exposure and internships.

- Offer opportunities to work alongside experienced pharmacists, observe pharmaceutical processes, and participate in patient care under supervision.

- Arrange internships in various settings, such as hospitals, retail pharmacies, pharmaceutical manufacturing, and regulatory bodies, to provide a well-rounded experiential learning.

9. Continuous Assessment and Progress Monitoring:

- Implement regular assessments, exams, and evaluations to track the progress of retraining pharmacists and identify areas needing improvement.

- Provide constructive feedback to help them understand their strengths and weaknesses, enabling them to work on their clinical skills and professional growth.

- Use data and feedback to adapt the program and address the evolving needs of the retraining pharmacists.

10. Networking and Collaboration:

- Establish a network of retraining pharmacists to foster collaboration, knowledge sharing, and peer support.

- Organize pharmacy conferences, webinars, and seminars to facilitate networking opportunities with healthcare professionals from various specialties and countries.

- Encourage retraining pharmacists to engage in research projects, publications, and quality improvement initiatives to contribute to the pharmacy community.

11. Program Evaluation and Improvement:

- Regularly evaluate the program's effectiveness through feedback from retraining pharmacists, mentors, and healthcare professionals.

- Analyze data and make necessary adjustments to the curriculum, teaching methodologies, and program structure to address emerging needs.

- Collaborate with local governments, healthcare organizations, and international partners to secure funding, resources, and support for program sustainability and expansion.

Implementing this comprehensive program would require collaboration with relevant stakeholders, including pharmacy schools, healthcare institutions, professional associations, and funding agencies. It is essential to ensure the availability of adequate resources, qualified trainers, and ongoing support to maximize the impact and success of the pharmacist retraining program.

Nursing and support Staff:

This is a comprehensive program to retrain nurses and support staff after uprising and victory in Iran who like many other professionals were admitted to professional schools based on religious or political connections rather than merit or aptitude:

Program Orientation and Needs Assessment:

- Conduct an orientation session to explain the program's objectives, expectations, and benefits to the nurses.

- Administer a comprehensive needs assessment to identify their individual strengths, weaknesses, and areas requiring improvement.

- Gather data on their nursing education background, clinical skills, and personal goals.

2. Core Nursing Knowledge Enhancement:

- Provide intensive training in core nursing knowledge, including anatomy, physiology, pharmacology, and nursing theories, to ensure a strong foundation.

- Offer specialized courses and workshops to update nurses on the latest nursing practices, evidence-based care, and global health issues.

- Utilize interactive teaching methods, case studies, and practical exercises to enhance critical thinking and clinical reasoning skills.

3. Clinical Skills Development:

- Conduct hands-on training sessions to improve clinical skills, including patient assessment, medication administration, wound care, and infection control.

- Provide simulated patient encounters and nursing simulations to practice and refine clinical skills in a controlled environment.

- Offer guidance on effective communication with patients, families, and healthcare teams, empathy, and cultural sensitivity to foster patient-centered care.

4. Specialized Training and Continuing Education:

- Develop specialized training modules based on the nurses' areas of interest or the healthcare needs of their communities.

- Offer continuing nursing education (CNE) courses, conferences, and workshops to keep the nurses updated with the latest nursing research, guidelines, and best practices.

- Collaborate with local and international nursing experts to deliver specialized training and share their expertise.

5. Ethical and Professional Development:

- Conduct sessions on nursing ethics, professional integrity, and patient advocacy to reinforce the importance of ethical conduct in nursing.

- Promote evidence-based nursing practice and encourage nurses to base their clinical decisions on scientific research and patient well-being.

- Facilitate discussions on the impact of religious or political influences on healthcare and emphasize the need for unbiased nursing care.

6. Mentoring and Individual Support:

- Assign experienced nurses as mentors to provide one-on-one guidance, support, and career advice to the retraining nurses.

- Conduct regular mentorship sessions to address individual concerns, monitor progress, and provide feedback on clinical skills and professional development.

- Encourage retraining nurses to seek advice and share experiences with their mentors, promoting a supportive learning environment.

7. Practical Exposure and Clinical Rotations:

- Collaborate with local healthcare institutions to provide practical exposure and clinical rotations in different healthcare settings.

- Offer opportunities to work alongside experienced nurses, observe procedures, and participate in patient care under supervision.

- Arrange rotations in various healthcare settings, such as hospitals, clinics, community health centers, and home care, to provide a well-rounded clinical experience.

8. Continuous Assessment and Progress Monitoring:

- Implement regular assessments, exams, and clinical evaluations to track the progress of retraining nurses and identify areas needing improvement.

- Provide constructive feedback to help them understand their strengths and weaknesses, enabling them to work on their clinical skills and professional growth.

- Use data and feedback to adapt the program and address the evolving needs of the retraining nurses.

9. Networking and Collaboration:

- Establish a network of retraining nurses to foster collaboration, knowledge sharing, and peer support.

- Organize nursing conferences, webinars, and seminars to facilitate networking opportunities with healthcare professionals from various specialties and countries.

- Encourage retraining nurses to engage in research projects, publications, and quality improvement initiatives to contribute to the nursing community.

10. Program Evaluation and Improvement:

- Regularly evaluate the program's effectiveness through feedback from retraining nurses, mentors, and healthcare professionals.

- Analyze data and make necessary adjustments to the curriculum, teaching methodologies, and program structure to address emerging needs.

- Collaborate with local governments, healthcare organizations, and international partners to secure funding, resources, and support for program sustainability and expansion.

Implementing this comprehensive program would require collaboration with relevant stakeholders, including nursing schools, healthcare institutions, professional associations, and funding agencies. It is essential to ensure the availability of adequate resources, qualified trainers, and ongoing support to maximize the impact and success of the nurse retraining program.

Practicing Physicians in different setting; Academic, private and government/charity sectors:

Program Orientation and Needs Assessment:

- Conduct an orientation session to explain the program's objectives, expectations, and benefits to the physicians.

- Administer a comprehensive needs assessment to identify their individual strengths, weaknesses, and areas requiring improvement.

- Gather data on their medical education background, clinical skills, and personal goals.

2. Core Medical Knowledge Enhancement:

- Provide intensive training in core medical knowledge, including anatomy, physiology, pharmacology, and pathology, to ensure a strong foundation.

- Offer specialized courses and workshops to update physicians on the latest medical advancements, evidence-based practices, and global health issues.

- Utilize interactive teaching methods, case studies, and practical exercises to enhance critical thinking and clinical reasoning skills.

3. Clinical Skills Development:

- Conduct hands-on training sessions to improve clinical skills, including history taking, physical examination, diagnosis, and treatment planning.

- Provide simulated patient encounters and medical simulations to practice and refine clinical skills in a controlled environment.

- Offer guidance on effective communication with patients, empathy, and cultural sensitivity to foster patient-centered care.

4. Specialized Training and Continuing Medical Education:

- Develop specialized training modules based on the physicians' areas of interest or the healthcare needs of their communities.

- Offer continuing medical education (CME) courses, conferences, and workshops to keep the physicians updated with the latest medical research, guidelines, and best practices.

- Collaborate with local and international medical experts to deliver specialized training and share their expertise.

5. Ethical and Professional Development:

- Conduct sessions on medical ethics, professional integrity, and patient confidentiality to reinforce the importance of ethical conduct in healthcare.

- Promote evidence-based medicine and encourage physicians to base their clinical decisions on scientific research and patient well-being.

- Facilitate discussions on the impact of religious or political influences on healthcare and emphasize the need for unbiased medical practice.

6. Mentoring and Individual Support:

- Assign experienced physicians as mentors to provide one-on-one guidance, support, and career advice to the retraining physicians.

- Conduct regular mentorship sessions to address individual concerns, monitor progress, and provide feedback on clinical skills and professional development.

- Encourage retraining physicians to seek advice and share experiences with their mentors, promoting a supportive learning environment.

7. Practical Exposure and Clinical Rotations:

- Collaborate with local healthcare institutions to provide practical exposure and clinical rotations in different medical specialties.

- Offer opportunities to work alongside experienced physicians, observe procedures, and participate in patient care under supervision.

- Arrange rotations in various healthcare settings, including hospitals, primary care clinics, and community health centers, to provide a well-rounded clinical experience.

8. Continuous Assessment and Progress Monitoring:

- Implement regular assessments, exams, and clinical evaluations to track the progress of retraining physicians and identify areas needing improvement.

- Provide constructive feedback to help them understand their strengths and weaknesses, enabling them to work on their clinical skills and professional growth.

- Use data and feedback to adapt the program and address the evolving needs of the retraining physicians.

9. Networking and Collaboration:

- Establish a network of retraining physicians to foster collaboration, knowledge sharing, and peer support.

- Organize medical conferences, webinars, and seminars to facilitate networking opportunities with healthcare professionals from various specialties and countries.

- Encourage retraining physicians to engage in research projects, publications, and quality improvement initiatives to contribute to the medical community.

10. Program Evaluation and Improvement:

- Regularly evaluate the program's effectiveness through feedback from retraining physicians, mentors, and healthcare professionals.

- Analyze data and make necessary adjustments to the curriculum, teaching methodologies, and program structure to address emerging needs.

- Collaborate with local governments, healthcare organizations, and international partners to secure funding, resources, and support for program sustainability and expansion.

Implementing this comprehensive program would require collaboration with relevant stakeholders, including medical institutions, professional associations, and funding agencies. It is crucial to ensure the availability of adequate resources, qualified trainers, and ongoing support to maximize the impact and success of the physician retraining program.

Mid Carrier practicing healthcare in different settings and specialties:

Program Orientation and Needs Assessment:

- Conduct an orientation session to explain the program's objectives, expectations, and benefits to the graduates.

- Administer a comprehensive needs assessment to identify their individual strengths, weaknesses, and areas requiring improvement.

- Gather data on their educational background, professional aspirations, and personal goals.

2. Remedial Education and Foundation Building:

- Provide remedial classes in fundamental subjects (e.g., mathematics, science, language skills) to fill knowledge gaps and ensure a strong foundation.

- Offer specialized courses to enhance critical thinking, problem-solving, and analytical skills necessary for their respective professions.

- Incorporate interactive teaching methods, practical exercises, and group discussions to engage and motivate the graduates.

3. Skill Enhancement and Professional Training:

- Develop a curriculum that focuses on the specific professional skills required in their field of study.

- Offer specialized courses and workshops to strengthen technical knowledge and practical competencies.

- Provide hands-on training, simulations, and real-life case studies to bridge the gap between theory and application.

- Collaborate with industry experts and professionals to deliver guest lectures, share practical insights, and offer guidance.

4. Ethical and Professional Development:

- Conduct sessions on professional ethics, integrity, and responsibility, emphasizing the importance of merit-based practices.

- Foster a culture of integrity, accountability, and transparency by promoting ethical decision-making and professional conduct.

- Organize workshops on effective communication, teamwork, and leadership skills to enhance their professional capabilities.

5. Mentoring and Individual Support:

- Assign mentors who are experienced professionals in their respective fields to provide personalized guidance and support.

- Conduct regular mentorship sessions to address individual concerns, monitor progress, and provide career guidance.

- Encourage graduates to seek advice and share experiences with their mentors, promoting a supportive learning environment.

6. Practical Exposure and Internships:

- Collaborate with local organizations, companies, and government bodies to provide practical exposure and internship opportunities.

- Facilitate internships, apprenticeships, or on-the-job training to enhance their practical skills and gain real-world experience.

- Encourage graduates to actively participate in community service initiatives, fostering a sense of social responsibility.

7. Continuous Assessment and Progress Monitoring:

- Implement regular assessments, exams, and performance evaluations to track their progress and identify areas needing improvement.

- Provide constructive feedback to help graduates understand their strengths and weaknesses, enabling them to work on their professional development.

- Use data and feedback to adapt the program and address the evolving needs of the graduates.

8. Networking and Alumni Engagement:

- Establish an alumni network to connect graduates with professionals, mentors, and peers in their field.

- Organize networking events, conferences, and seminars to facilitate knowledge sharing and professional connections.

- Encourage alumni to contribute back to the program by mentoring new participants or providing guest lectures.

9. Continuous Learning and Growth:

- Emphasize the importance of lifelong learning and professional development to ensure graduates stay updated with industry trends.

- Provide resources, access to online courses, and learning materials to support their ongoing growth and skill enhancement.

- Encourage graduates to pursue higher education, research opportunities, or certifications to further advance in their careers.

10. Program Evaluation and Improvement:

- Regularly evaluate the program's effectiveness through feedback from graduates, mentors, and industry professionals.

- Analyze data and make necessary adjustments to the curriculum, teaching methodologies, and program structure.

- Collaborate with stakeholders to secure funding, resources, and support for program sustainability and expansion.

Remember, this comprehensive program outline serves as a starting point, and the actual implementation would require thorough planning, collaboration with relevant organizations, and securing necessary resources.

Rebuilding Iran: Government in Exile

To establish a shadow governance structure that undermines the credibility of the unpopular government and the faction, a cabinet in exile can take several steps. Here are some approaches they can consider:

1. Develop Policy Platforms: The cabinet in exile should develop comprehensive policy platforms that address the needs and aspirations of the people. These platforms should outline clear and practical solutions to the challenges faced by the country. By presenting well-thought-out policies, the cabinet in exile can demonstrate their competence and ability to govern effectively.

2. Formulate Strategic Plans: The cabinet in exile should formulate strategic plans that outline their vision for the future and the steps needed to achieve it. These plans should include specific goals, timelines, and action items. By presenting a detailed roadmap for progress, the cabinet in exile can showcase their commitment to building a better future for the country.

3. Provide Essential Services: The cabinet in exile can focus on providing essential services to the population within their capacity. This can include healthcare, education, infrastructure development, and economic support. By demonstrating their ability to meet the needs of the people, the cabinet in exile can undermine the credibility of the unpopular government and the faction, which may be failing to provide adequate services.

4. Foster Transparency and Accountability: The cabinet in exile should prioritize transparency and accountability in their governance structure. They should establish mechanisms for monitoring and reporting on their activities, ensuring that resources are used effectively, and corruption is minimized. By showcasing a commitment to transparency and accountability, the cabinet in exile can contrast themselves with the unpopular government and the faction, which may be characterized by corruption and lack of transparency.

5. Engage with Local Communities: The cabinet in exile should actively engage with local communities to understand their needs and concerns. They can hold town hall meetings, community forums, or establish local committees to involve the population in decision-making processes. By actively involving the people, the cabinet in exile can demonstrate their commitment to participatory governance and contrast themselves with the unpopular government and the faction, which may be disconnected from the needs of the people.

6. Promote Rule of Law: The cabinet in exile should prioritize promoting the rule of law and protecting human rights. They should establish mechanisms to ensure the fair and impartial administration of justice, protect civil liberties, and safeguard the rights of the population. By upholding the rule of law, the cabinet in exile can contrast themselves with the faction, which may be engaged in human rights abuses and disregard for the law.
7. Build International Partnerships: The cabinet in exile should actively seek international partnerships and support for their governance initiatives. They can engage with international organizations, foreign governments, and civil society groups to garner recognition and assistance. By securing international support, the cabinet in exile can gain legitimacy and demonstrate their capacity to govern effectively.
8. Communicate Effectively: The cabinet in exile should invest in effective communication strategies to disseminate their policies, achievements, and vision to the population and the international community. They can utilize various communication channels, including social media, traditional media, and public events, to engage with the public and build credibility. By effectively communicating their message, the cabinet in exile can counter the narratives of the unpopular government and the faction.
9. It is important for the cabinet in exile to continuously assess and adapt their strategies based on the evolving situation. They should also seek input and feedback from the population to ensure that their shadow governance structure reflects the needs and aspirations of the people.

Setting up a government in exile with a full cabinet function is a complex process that requires careful planning and consideration. Here are the key steps involved:

1. Define the Purpose: Clearly articulate the purpose and objectives of the government in exile. This will guide the decision-making process and help in forming the cabinet.
2. Formulate a Structure: Determine the structure and composition of the cabinet. Identify the key ministerial positions that need to be filled, such as defense, finance, foreign affairs, etc. Consider the expertise and experience required for each position.
3. Identify Potential Cabinet Members: Identify individuals who are willing to serve in the cabinet and possess the necessary skills and knowledge. Look for individuals with relevant experience in government, diplomacy, or other relevant fields.
4. Assign Roles and Responsibilities: Once the cabinet members are identified, assign specific roles and responsibilities to each minister based on their expertise and the needs of the government in exile.
5. Establish Communication Channels: Set up effective communication channels to facilitate coordination and decision-making among the cabinet members. This can include regular virtual meetings, email communication, or other secure platforms.

6. Develop Policy Framework: Work collectively with the cabinet members to develop a policy framework that outlines the government's priorities and strategies. This will guide the decision-making process and provide a basis for governance.
7. Engage with International Partners: Reach out to international partners, governments, and organizations to seek recognition and support for the government in exile. This involves diplomatic efforts and building alliances to advance the cause.
8. Mobilize Resources: Identify and mobilize the necessary resources, such as funding, personnel, and logistical support, to sustain the functioning of the government in exile. This may involve seeking financial assistance from international partners or engaging with diaspora communities.
9. Advocate for the Cause: Utilize various platforms and channels to advocate for the cause of the government in exile. This can include media engagements, public diplomacy, and lobbying efforts to garner support and raise awareness.
10. Adapt and Evolve: Continuously adapt and evolve the functioning of the government in exile based on changing circumstances and challenges. Regularly review and assess the effectiveness of the cabinet and make necessary adjustments as required.

Remember, setting up a government in exile is a complex and dynamic process. It requires strong leadership, strategic thinking, and the ability to adapt to changing circumstances.

Setting up a government in exile involves several key steps.

Proposed Steps:

1. Leadership and Representation: Identify a leader or figurehead who will represent the government in exile. This person should have the credibility and support of the exiled community.
2. Constituent Assembly: Establish a constituent assembly comprising representatives from different political, social, and ethnic groups. This assembly will serve as the primary decision-making body for the government in exile.
3. Legal Framework: Develop a legal framework that outlines the structure, functions, and powers of the government in exile. This framework should be in line with international law and the principles of democracy.
4. Cabinet Formation: Form a cabinet with key ministerial positions such as defense, foreign affairs, finance, and justice. Select individuals who have the necessary expertise and experience to handle these roles effectively.
5. Government Departments: Establish various government departments to handle specific areas of governance, such as education, healthcare, infrastructure, and economy. These departments will be responsible for implementing policies and providing services.

6. Diplomatic Engagement: Engage with international partners, governments, and organizations to seek recognition and support for the government in exile. This involves diplomatic efforts, building alliances, and advocating for the cause.
7. Resource Mobilization: Identify and mobilize the necessary resources to sustain the functioning of the government in exile. This includes financial resources, personnel, and logistical support. Seek funding from international partners or engage with diaspora communities.
8. Communication and Outreach: Establish effective communication channels to disseminate information and engage with the exiled community, international partners, and the general public. This can include websites, social media platforms, and regular updates.
9. Legal and Human Rights Advocacy: Advocate for the rights and well-being of the exiled community through legal and human rights channels. Raise awareness about the situation and seek international support for addressing any violations or injustices.
10. Transition Planning: Develop a comprehensive plan for the transition to a post-conflict or post-oppression scenario. This includes preparing for the return of the government to the home country and managing the transitional period effectively.
11. Remember, setting up a government in exile is a complex and challenging process. It requires careful planning, coordination, and engagement with various stakeholders. Adaptation and flexibility are crucial as the situation evolves.

Establishing a legal framework that aligns with international law and democratic principles is important for several reasons:

1. Legitimacy: A government in exile seeks to gain legitimacy and recognition from the international community. By adhering to international law and democratic principles, the government in exile demonstrates its commitment to upholding human rights, the rule of law, and democratic governance. This enhances its credibility and increases the likelihood of gaining recognition and support from other countries.
2. Accountability: A legal framework based on international law and democratic principles establishes clear guidelines and mechanisms for accountability. It ensures that the government in exile operates within the bounds of legality and is subject to checks and balances. This fosters transparency, prevents abuse of power, and promotes good governance.
3. Protection of Human Rights: International law and democratic principles prioritize the protection of human rights. By aligning with these principles, a government in exile demonstrates its commitment to upholding and safeguarding the rights and freedoms of its citizens. This includes protecting individuals from arbitrary detention, torture, and other human rights abuses.

4. International Cooperation: Adhering to international law and democratic principles facilitates cooperation and engagement with other countries and international organizations. It creates a common framework for collaboration, negotiation, and the resolution of disputes. This enables the government in exile to establish diplomatic relationships, seek support, and advocate for its cause on the global stage.
5. Transitional Justice: A legal framework based on international law and democratic principles provides a basis for transitional justice processes. It allows for the investigation, prosecution, and accountability for human rights violations and atrocities committed by the previous regime. This promotes reconciliation, justice, and the restoration of trust in the government.
6. Stability and Peacebuilding: A government in exile that operates within the framework of international law and democratic principles contributes to stability and peacebuilding efforts. By promoting inclusivity, respect for human rights, and democratic governance, it lays the foundation for a peaceful and just society in the future.

In summary, establishing a legal framework that aligns with international law and democratic principles enhances the legitimacy, accountability, and credibility of a government in exile. It ensures the protection of human rights, facilitates international cooperation, supports transitional justice, and promotes stability and peacebuilding.

Aligning with international law and democratic principles contributes to stability and peacebuilding efforts for a government in exile in several ways:

1. Legitimacy and Recognition: By adhering to international law and democratic principles, a government in exile gains legitimacy and recognition from the international community. This legitimacy enhances its standing and credibility, making it more likely to receive support and assistance from other countries. This recognition helps to stabilize the government in exile and provides a foundation for peacebuilding efforts.
2. Conflict Resolution: International law and democratic principles emphasize peaceful conflict resolution through negotiation, mediation, and diplomacy. By adopting these principles, a government in exile demonstrates its commitment to resolving conflicts through peaceful means rather than resorting to violence. This can help de-escalate tensions and create an environment conducive to stability and peacebuilding.
3. Inclusivity and Participation: Democratic principles promote inclusivity and the participation of all stakeholders in decision-making processes. Involving diverse groups in the government in exile, ensures that different voices and perspectives are heard and considered. Inclusion and participation help to address grievances, build trust, and promote a sense of ownership among the exiled community. This

can contribute to stability and peacebuilding by reducing divisions and fostering a sense of unity.

4. Protection of Human Rights: International law and democratic principles prioritize the protection of human rights. By aligning with these principles, a government in exile demonstrates its commitment to upholding and safeguarding the rights and freedoms of its citizens. This includes protecting individuals from human rights abuses, promoting equality, and ensuring access to justice. The protection of human rights is crucial for creating a stable and peaceful society.

5. Transitional Justice: Aligning with international law and democratic principles provides a basis for transitional justice processes. Transitional justice seeks to address past human rights abuses, promote accountability, and facilitate reconciliation. By establishing mechanisms for truth-seeking, justice, reparations, and institutional reforms, a government in exile can contribute to healing wounds, promoting reconciliation, and building a foundation for sustainable peace.

6. Good Governance: Adhering to democratic principles fosters good governance practices, such as transparency, accountability, and the rule of law. These principles help to combat corruption, ensure effective service delivery, and promote public trust in the government. Good governance contributes to stability and peacebuilding by creating an environment of predictability, fairness, and legitimacy.

In summary, aligning with international law and democratic principles enhances the legitimacy, inclusivity, and accountability of a government in exile. It promotes peaceful conflict resolution, protects human rights, supports transitional justice, and fosters good governance. These factors collectively contribute to stability and peacebuilding efforts, laying the groundwork for a peaceful and prosperous future for the exiled community.

The involvement of diverse groups in decision-making processes contributes to stability and peacebuilding for a government in exile in the following ways:

1. Inclusivity and Representation: When diverse groups are involved in decision-making processes, it ensures that different perspectives, interests, and concerns are considered. Inclusion helps to address grievances and reduce feelings of exclusion or marginalization among various segments of the exiled community. When people feel represented and included, it fosters a sense of ownership, belonging, and legitimacy, which are essential for stability and peacebuilding.

2. Conflict Resolution: Involving diverse groups in decision-making processes allows for the peaceful resolution of conflicts. By bringing together representatives from different factions or communities, discussions can take place, grievances can be aired, and compromises can be reached. This process helps to build trust, bridge divides, and find mutually acceptable solutions. Inclusive decision-making can contribute to the de-escalation of tensions and the prevention or mitigation of conflicts within the exiled community.

3. Social Cohesion and Unity: The involvement of diverse groups in decision-making processes helps to foster social cohesion and unity. When people from different backgrounds, ethnicities, religions, or political affiliations participate in decision-making, it promotes interaction, understanding, and empathy. It creates opportunities for dialogue, collaboration, and the building of relationships across divides. This sense of unity and shared purpose strengthens social bonds and contributes to stability and peacebuilding.
4. Sustainable Solutions: Inclusive decision-making processes tend to lead to more sustainable solutions. When diverse groups are involved, a wider range of perspectives, knowledge, and expertise is considered. This diversity of input can lead to more comprehensive and innovative solutions that address the root causes of conflicts or challenges. Sustainable solutions are more likely to be accepted and implemented by the exiled community, contributing to long-term stability and peace.
5. Empowerment and Participation: Involving diverse groups in decision-making processes empowers individuals and communities by giving them a voice and the opportunity to shape their future. When people feel empowered and can participate in decision-making, it increases their stake in the peacebuilding process. This sense of agency and participation fosters a sense of responsibility and commitment to maintaining peace and stability.
6. Reconciliation and Trust-Building: Inclusive decision-making processes create spaces for dialogue, reconciliation, and trust-building among diverse groups. It allows for the acknowledgment of past grievances, the airing of concerns, and the opportunity for dialogue and understanding. Through inclusive decision-making, bridges can be built between different factions or communities, promoting social healing, reconciliation, and the building of trust.

In summary, the involvement of diverse groups in decision-making processes promotes inclusivity, representation, conflict resolution, social cohesion, sustainable solutions, empowerment, and reconciliation. These factors collectively contribute to stability and peacebuilding for a government in exile by addressing grievances, building trust, fostering unity, and creating a sense of ownership and shared responsibility for peace.

The participation of people from different backgrounds, ethnicities, religions, or political affiliations in decision-making processes contributes to social cohesion and unity in the following ways:

1. Representation and Inclusivity: When people from diverse backgrounds participate in decision-making processes, it ensures that a wide range of perspectives, interests, and concerns are taken into account. This representation and inclusivity create a sense of belonging and ownership among different groups within the society. When individuals see themselves represented in the decision-making process, it fosters a greater sense of unity and shared purpose.

2. Cross-Cultural Understanding: The participation of people from different backgrounds promotes cross-cultural understanding and empathy. Through engagement in decision-making, individuals can learn about and appreciate the perspectives, values, and experiences of others. This understanding helps to break down stereotypes, reduce prejudice, and build bridges between diverse groups. It fosters a sense of unity based on shared humanity and respect for diversity.
3. Collaboration and Cooperation: Decision-making processes that involve people from different backgrounds foster collaboration and cooperation. By bringing together individuals with different skills, knowledge, and experiences, it encourages the sharing of ideas, expertise, and resources. This collaboration leads to innovative and comprehensive solutions that address the needs and aspirations of diverse groups. Working together towards common goals builds a sense of unity and collective responsibility.
4. Conflict Resolution and Mediation: The participation of people from different backgrounds in decision-making processes provides an opportunity for peaceful conflict resolution and mediation. When individuals with diverse perspectives and interests come together, they have a chance to engage in dialogue, negotiate, and find mutually acceptable solutions. This process helps to bridge divides, build trust, and address grievances, contributing to social cohesion and unity.
5. Social Integration and Inclusion: The participation of people from different backgrounds in decision-making processes promotes social integration and inclusion. When individuals from marginalized or underrepresented groups have a seat at the table, it challenges existing power imbalances and promotes equal opportunities. This inclusion helps to break down barriers, reduce social exclusion, and create a sense of belonging and unity within society.
6. Shared Responsibility and Ownership: When people from different backgrounds participate in decision-making processes, it fosters a sense of shared responsibility and ownership for the well-being of the community. This shared responsibility encourages individuals to work together towards common goals, fostering a sense of unity and solidarity. It creates a collective sense of ownership over the decisions made, leading to greater commitment and implementation of those decisions.

In summary, the participation of people from different backgrounds, ethnicities, religions, or political affiliations in decision-making processes promotes social cohesion and unity by ensuring representation, fostering cross-cultural understanding, encouraging collaboration, facilitating conflict resolution, promoting social integration, and creating a sense of shared responsibility and ownership. These factors collectively contribute to a more cohesive and unified society.

Forming Governing Body: Cabinet vs Council in Exile:

The structure of a government in exile can vary depending on the specific circumstances and goals of the exiled government. However, there are common elements that are often found in the structure of a government in exile. Here is a general outline of the structure:

1. Head of State: The government in exile typically has a recognized leader who serves as the head of state. This leader may be the president, prime minister, or another designated individual who represents the exiled government and its interests.
2. Cabinet or Council of Ministers: The government in exile usually has a cabinet or council of ministers who are responsible for specific portfolios or areas of governance. These ministers are appointed by the head of state and are responsible for overseeing various government functions such as foreign affairs, defense, finance, and justice.
3. Legislative Body: In some cases, a government in exile may have a legislative body or parliament that represents the exiled population and is responsible for making laws and policies. The legislative body may be elected or appointed by the exiled community and serves as a forum for debate, decision-making, and representation.
4. Diplomatic Corps: A government in exile often maintains a diplomatic corps, which represents the exiled government and engages with international actors, governments, and organizations. The diplomatic corps works to build alliances, advocate for the interests of the exiled government, and seek support for the cause of the exiled community.
5. Administrative Departments: The government in exile may have various administrative departments or agencies responsible for specific areas of governance, such as finance, defense, foreign affairs, and humanitarian assistance. These departments help implement government policies and provide services to the exiled community.
6. Advisory Councils and Committees: A government in exile may establish advisory councils or committees composed of experts, community leaders, and representatives from different sectors to provide advice and recommendations on various issues. These advisory bodies help inform decision-making and ensure diverse perspectives are considered.
7. Support Networks and Institutions: A government in exile often establishes support networks and institutions to aid and services to the exiled community. These may include healthcare services, education programs, legal aid, and social support networks to address the needs of the exiled population.
8. It's important to note that the structure of a government in exile can evolve and may be influenced by factors such as the size of the exiled community, the level of recognition from the international community, and the specific goals and challenges faced by the exiled government.

The cabinet or council of ministers in a government in exile has various responsibilities, which can vary depending on the specific circumstances and goals of the exiled government. However, some common responsibilities of the cabinet or council of ministers in a government in exile include:

1. Policy Formulation: The cabinet or council of ministers is responsible for formulating policies and strategies that align with the goals and objectives of the exiled government. They analyze the political, economic, and social situation and develop plans to address the needs and aspirations of the exiled community.
2. Governance and Administration: The cabinet or council of ministers oversees the governance and administration of the exiled government. They establish and implement rules and regulations, manage government resources, and ensure the smooth functioning of government institutions and departments.
3. Portfolio Management: Each minister in the cabinet or council is assigned a specific portfolio or area of governance. They are responsible for managing and overseeing the functions, policies, and programs related to their respective portfolios. For example, there may be ministers for foreign affairs, defense, finance, justice, education, health, and other key sectors.
4. Decision-Making: The cabinet or council of ministers engages in collective decision-making. They discuss and deliberate on important matters, review proposals and recommendations, and make decisions that impact the exiled government and its community. These decisions may include foreign policy positions, resource allocation, legislation, and other significant issues.
5. Coordination and Collaboration: The cabinet or council of ministers works collaboratively to ensure coordination and coherence in the implementation of government policies and programs. They communicate and cooperate, share information and resources, and coordinate efforts across different portfolios to achieve common objectives.
6. Representation and Advocacy: The cabinet or council of ministers represents the exiled government in interactions with the international community, governments, organizations, and other stakeholders. They advocate for the interests of the exiled community, seek support for the cause of the exiled government, and build alliances to advance their goals.
7. Communication and Public Engagement: The cabinet or council of ministers communicates government policies, decisions, and initiatives to the exiled community and the public. They engage with the media, issue statements, and participate in public events to inform and involve the exiled population, seek feedback, and address their concerns.

8. Crisis Management: In times of crisis or emergency, the cabinet or council of ministers takes a leadership role in managing the situation. They develop contingency plans, coordinate response efforts, and provide guidance and support to the exiled community to ensure their safety, well-being, and resilience.

It's important to note that the specific responsibilities of the cabinet or council of ministers in a government in exile can be influenced by factors such as the size of the exiled community, the level of recognition from the international community, and the specific goals and challenges faced by the exiled government.

Governing Body in Transition and During Crisis:

In times of crisis or emergency, the cabinet or council of ministers in a government in exile assumes several key tasks to effectively manage the situation and ensure the well-being of the exiled community. Some of these tasks include:

1. Crisis Assessment and Planning: The cabinet or council of ministers assesses the nature and severity of the crisis or emergency. They gather information, analyze the impact on the exiled community, and develop a comprehensive crisis response plan. This plan outlines the necessary actions, resource allocation, and coordination mechanisms to mitigate the crisis and protect the interests of the exiled community.
2. Decision-Making and Policy Direction: The cabinet or council of ministers makes critical decisions and provides policy direction during the crisis. They evaluate available options, consult with experts, and determine the best course of action to address the immediate and long-term needs of the exiled community. This may involve activating emergency protocols, implementing measures for safety and security, and adapting government policies to the evolving crisis.
3. Coordination and Collaboration: The cabinet or council of ministers takes the lead in coordinating and collaborating with relevant stakeholders, both within the exiled government and externally. They work closely with emergency response agencies, humanitarian organizations, and other governments to ensure a coordinated and effective response. This includes sharing information, pooling resources, and coordinating efforts to provide essential services, support, and assistance to the affected population.
4. Resource Management: During a crisis or emergency, the cabinet or council of ministers manages and allocates resources to address the immediate needs of the exiled community. This involves assessing available resources, mobilizing additional support, and prioritizing resource allocation based on the severity and urgency of the situation. They may coordinate the distribution of food, water, shelter, medical supplies, and other necessary provisions to those affected by the crisis.
5. Communication and Public Engagement: The cabinet or council of ministers plays a crucial role in communicating timely and accurate information to the exiled

community and the public. They provide regular updates, issue statements, and use various communication channels to disseminate important information about the crisis, government response efforts, and safety measures. They also engage with the media, conduct press briefings, and address public concerns to maintain transparency and build trust during the crisis.

6. Crisis Mitigation and Recovery: The cabinet or council of ministers focuses on mitigating the impact of the crisis and facilitating the recovery of the exiled community. They implement measures to ensure the safety and well-being of the population, including emergency healthcare services, psychological support, and social assistance programs. They also develop strategies for long-term recovery, such as rebuilding infrastructure, revitalizing the economy, and restoring normalcy in the aftermath of the crisis.

7. International Advocacy and Support: During a crisis or emergency, the cabinet or council of ministers advocates for international support and assistance. They engage with the international community, humanitarian organizations, and other governments to seek aid, resources, and expertise to effectively manage the crisis and provide relief to the affected population. They may also work towards raising awareness about the crisis and advocating for the rights and needs of the exiled community on the global stage.

It's important to note that the specific tasks of the cabinet or council of ministers in a government in exile during a crisis or emergency can vary depending on the nature and scale of the crisis, the available resources, and the unique circumstances of the exiled government and community.

Immediate Relief and Chaos Management:

The cabinet or council of ministers in a government in exile implements various measures to provide immediate relief to the affected population during a crisis. Some of these measures include:

1. Emergency Food Distribution: The cabinet or council of ministers coordinates the distribution of food to ensure that the affected population has access to an adequate and nutritious supply. They establish distribution centers, work with local organizations and humanitarian agencies, and mobilize resources to provide food assistance to those in need.

2. Water and Sanitation Services: The cabinet or council of ministers ensures access to clean water and sanitation facilities for the affected population. They establish temporary water supply systems, distribute water purification tablets or equipment, and support the construction or repair of sanitation facilities to prevent the spread of diseases.

3. Shelter and Emergency Housing: The cabinet or council of ministers addresses the immediate housing needs of the affected population. They provide temporary shelter options such as tents, emergency shelters, or communal centers. They may also coordinate with humanitarian organizations or local authorities to secure safe and suitable shelter for those displaced by the crisis.
4. Medical Assistance and Healthcare: The cabinet or council of ministers focuses on providing immediate medical assistance and healthcare services to the affected population. They establish emergency healthcare facilities, deploy medical personnel, and ensure the availability of essential medical supplies and equipment. They may also coordinate medical evacuations for those in critical condition.
5. Psychological Support and Counseling: The cabinet or council of ministers recognizes the importance of psychological support during a crisis. They establish counseling services or collaborate with mental health organizations to provide emotional support and counseling to individuals and families affected by the crisis. This helps address trauma, anxiety, and other psychological impacts of the crisis.
6. Emergency Cash Assistance: The cabinet or council of ministers may provide emergency cash assistance to vulnerable individuals and families affected by the crisis. This helps meet immediate needs and enables the affected population to access essential goods and services.
7. Communication and Information Dissemination: The cabinet or council of ministers ensures effective communication and information dissemination to the affected population. They utilize various channels, such as public announcements, radio broadcasts, or mobile messaging, to provide updates on relief efforts, safety instructions, and available support services.
8. Protection and Safety Measures: The cabinet or council of ministers takes measures to ensure the protection and safety of the affected population. They work with law enforcement agencies or establish security mechanisms to prevent looting, exploitation, or other forms of harm. They may also initiate measures to reunite separated families or provide special protection for vulnerable groups such as children, women, or the elderly.

It's important to note that the specific measures implemented by the cabinet or council of ministers to provide immediate relief to the affected population can vary depending on the nature and scale of the crisis, the available resources, and the unique circumstances of the exiled government and community.

Outside and Inside Bridge:

The cabinet or council of ministers in a government in exile implements various measures to provide immediate relief to the affected population during a crisis. Some of these measures include:

1. Emergency Food Distribution: The cabinet or council of ministers coordinates the distribution of food to ensure that the affected population has access to an adequate and nutritious supply. They establish distribution centers, work with local organizations and humanitarian agencies, and mobilize resources to provide food assistance to those in need.
2. Water and Sanitation Services: The cabinet or council of ministers ensures access to clean water and sanitation facilities for the affected population. They establish temporary water supply systems, distribute water purification tablets or equipment, and support the construction or repair of sanitation facilities to prevent the spread of diseases.
3. Shelter and Emergency Housing: The cabinet or council of ministers addresses the immediate housing needs of the affected population. They provide temporary shelter options such as tents, emergency shelters, or communal centers. They may also coordinate with humanitarian organizations or local authorities to secure safe and suitable shelter for those displaced by the crisis.
4. Medical Assistance and Healthcare: The cabinet or council of ministers focuses on providing immediate medical assistance and healthcare services to the affected population. They establish emergency healthcare facilities, deploy medical personnel, and ensure the availability of essential medical supplies and equipment. They may also coordinate medical evacuations for those in critical condition.
5. Psychological Support and Counseling: The cabinet or council of ministers recognizes the importance of psychological support during a crisis. They establish counseling services or collaborate with mental health organizations to provide emotional support and counseling to individuals and families affected by the crisis. This helps address trauma, anxiety, and other psychological impacts of the crisis.
6. Emergency Cash Assistance: The cabinet or council of ministers may provide emergency cash assistance to vulnerable individuals and families affected by the crisis. This helps meet immediate needs and enables the affected population to access essential goods and services.
7. Communication and Information Dissemination: The cabinet or council of ministers ensures effective communication and information dissemination to the affected population. They utilize various channels, such as public announcements, radio broadcasts, or mobile messaging, to provide updates on relief efforts, safety instructions, and available support services.
8. Protection and Safety Measures: The cabinet or council of ministers takes measures to ensure the protection and safety of the affected population. They work with law enforcement agencies or establish security mechanisms to prevent looting, exploitation, or other forms of harm. They may also initiate measures to reunite separated families or provide special protection for vulnerable groups such as children, women, or the elderly.

It's important to note that the specific measures implemented by the cabinet or council of ministers to provide immediate relief to the affected population can vary depending on the nature and scale of the crisis, the available resources, and the unique circumstances of the exiled government and community.

Political and current government engagement:

The cabinet or council in exile utilizes diplomatic channels to engage with the target country's government in several ways:

1. Diplomatic Missions: The cabinet or council in exile may establish diplomatic missions or embassies in countries that have recognized their legitimacy or are sympathetic to their cause. These diplomatic missions serve as official channels of communication and representation, allowing the cabinet or council to engage directly with the target country's government.
2. Diplomatic Notes and Letters: The cabinet or council in exile can send diplomatic notes or letters to the target country's government, expressing their concerns, stating their positions, or requesting meetings or dialogue. These diplomatic communications are formal and carry diplomatic weight, conveying the cabinet or council's official stance on various issues.
3. Diplomatic Meetings and Negotiations: The cabinet or council in exile may request and participate in diplomatic meetings and negotiations with the target country's government. These meetings can provide an opportunity to discuss matters of mutual interest, address concerns, and explore potential areas of cooperation or resolution.
4. Diplomatic Recognition: The cabinet or council in exile seeks diplomatic recognition from other countries, which can indirectly influence the target country's government. When other countries recognize the legitimacy of the cabinet or council, it can increase their credibility and strengthen their position when engaging with the target country's government.
5. Diplomatic Lobbying: The cabinet or council in exile engages in diplomatic lobbying efforts to gain support from other countries, including those with influence over the target country's government. They may seek the assistance of friendly governments, engage in diplomatic negotiations, or participate in international forums to advocate for their cause and garner diplomatic support.
6. Track II Diplomacy: In situations where direct diplomatic engagement with the target country's government is challenging or not possible, the cabinet or council in exile may engage in track II diplomacy. This involves unofficial dialogues and negotiations between non-governmental entities, such as think tanks, academics, or civil society organizations, to explore potential solutions and build relationships that can indirectly influence the target country's government.

7. International Organizations: The cabinet or council in exile can utilize international organizations, such as the United Nations or regional bodies, to engage with the target country's government. They may participate in diplomatic conferences, submit reports or petitions, or seek the assistance of international mediators or envoys to facilitate dialogue and resolution of conflicts.
8. It's important to note that the effectiveness of diplomatic channels in engaging with the target country's government can vary depending on various factors, including the political landscape, international relations, and the willingness of the target country's government to engage with the cabinet or council in exile.

Hostile Government and Hostility Management:

The cabinet or council in exile faces significant challenges when dealing with a target country that has a hostile government. To mitigate subversion and facilitate a transition in such a situation, they can employ several strategies:

1. International Support: The cabinet or council in exile seeks international support from other countries, international organizations, and influential individuals. They engage in diplomatic efforts, attend international conferences or forums, and build alliances with other exiled governments or organizations to amplify their voice and garner support for their cause. International support can exert pressure on the hostile government and provide leverage for the cabinet or council in exile to negotiate for a peaceful transition.
2. Advocacy and Public Awareness: The cabinet or council in exile engages in advocacy and public awareness campaigns to raise awareness about their cause and garner support within the target country and internationally. They utilize various media platforms, social networks, and public events to highlight human rights abuses, political repression, and the need for a peaceful transition in the target country. By mobilizing public opinion, they can put pressure on the hostile government and create momentum for change.
3. Nonviolent Resistance: The cabinet or council in exile promotes nonviolent resistance as a means to challenge the hostile government's authority and mobilize the population. They encourage peaceful protests, civil disobedience, and acts of resistance that demonstrate the people's desire for change. Nonviolent resistance can help to delegitimize the hostile government and create an environment conducive to a peaceful transition.
4. External Diplomatic Pressure: The cabinet or council in exile works to build alliances with friendly governments and international organizations that can exert diplomatic pressure on the hostile government. They seek economic sanctions, travel bans, arms embargoes, and other measures to isolate and weaken the hostile government. External diplomatic pressure can increase the cost of maintaining power for the hostile government and create opportunities for a negotiated transition.

5. Track II Diplomacy and Dialogue: The cabinet or council in exile engages in track II diplomacy, which involves unofficial dialogues and negotiations between non-governmental entities, to explore potential solutions and build relationships. They may engage with influential individuals, civil society organizations, or think tanks within the target country to foster dialogue, bridge divides, and find common ground for a peaceful transition.
6. Support for Civil Society: The cabinet or council in exile provides support to civil society organizations and activists within the target country. They offer resources, training, and protection to those working to promote democracy, human rights, and a peaceful transition. Supporting civil society strengthens the local movement for change and helps to undermine the hostile government's control.
7. International Legal Mechanisms: The cabinet or council in exile utilizes international legal mechanisms to hold the hostile government accountable for human rights abuses and political repression. They may submit reports to international courts or seek investigations into human rights violations. International legal mechanisms can help to expose the actions of the hostile government and create pressure for a transition.

It's important to note that mitigating subversion and facilitating a transition in a target country with a hostile government is a complex and challenging process. The specific strategies employed by the cabinet or council in exile will depend on the unique circumstances and dynamics of the situation.

Engaging Communities and Citizen Awareness:

The cabinet or council in exile can use several methods to raise awareness and garner support for their cause:

1. Media Engagement: The cabinet or council in exile can engage with local and international media outlets to amplify their message and raise awareness about their cause. They can issue press releases, give interviews, publish articles, or organize press conferences to share their perspectives, highlight human rights abuses, and advocate for a peaceful transition. Utilizing media platforms helps to reach a wider audience and generate public attention.

2. Social media and Online Activism: The cabinet or council in exile can leverage social media platforms and online activism to engage with a global audience and mobilize support. They can create official social media accounts, share updates, videos, and infographics, and encourage supporters to share their content. Online campaigns, hashtags, and petitions can help to raise awareness, engage with supporters, and put pressure on the hostile government.

3. Public Events and Demonstrations: The cabinet or council in exile can organize public events, demonstrations, and rallies to gather support and create visibility for their cause.

These events can include speeches, cultural performances, or symbolic acts that draw attention to their plight. Public events provide an opportunity to engage directly with supporters, media, and the general public, generating momentum and solidarity.

4. Advocacy with International Organizations: The cabinet or council in exile can engage with international organizations, such as the United Nations, regional bodies, or human rights organizations, to advocate for their cause. They can submit reports, petitions, or appeals, participate in relevant conferences or forums, and engage with international envoys or mediators. Advocacy with international organizations can help raise the profile of their cause and put pressure on the hostile government.

5. Engaging with Diaspora Communities: The cabinet or council in exile can engage with diaspora communities from the target country residing in other parts of the world. They can organize events, meetings, or conferences to connect with diaspora communities, share updates, and seek their support. Diaspora communities often maintain strong ties to their home country and can be influential in raising awareness and mobilizing support.

6. Collaboration with Civil Society Organizations: The cabinet or council in exile can collaborate with local and international civil society organizations that share their goals and values. They can form partnerships, participate in joint campaigns, or support initiatives that promote democracy, human rights, and a peaceful transition. Collaboration with civil society organizations helps to expand their network, gain credibility, and reach wider audiences.

7. Cultural Diplomacy: The cabinet or council in exile can utilize cultural diplomacy to raise awareness and garner support. They can organize cultural events, art exhibitions, film screenings, or concerts that reflect the rich cultural heritage of the target country. Cultural diplomacy helps to engage people on an emotional level, fostering understanding and empathy for the cause.

8. Engaging with Academia and Think Tanks: The cabinet or council in exile can engage with academics, researchers, and think tanks to generate research, analysis, and policy recommendations related to their cause. They can organize conferences, seminars, or lectures that bring together experts and policymakers to discuss the situation in the target country. Engaging with academia and think tanks helps to build intellectual support and shape the narrative around their cause.

It's important for the cabinet or council in exile to adapt their strategies based on the specific context, target audience, and available resources. A multifaceted approach that combines various methods can maximize their impact and generate sustained support for their cause.

Resource Optimizations:

Adapting strategies based on the specific context, target audience, and available resources is important for the cabinet or council in exile for several reasons:

1. Relevance and Effectiveness: Different contexts and target audiences may respond differently to various outreach methods. Adapting strategies allows the cabinet or council in exile to tailor their approach to the specific circumstances and preferences of the target audience. By understanding the local context and the needs of the audience, they can design strategies that resonate and have a greater chance of being effective in raising awareness and garnering support.

2. Cultural Sensitivity: Adapting strategies based on the specific context helps ensure cultural sensitivity. Different cultures may have different norms, values, and communication styles. By taking these cultural factors into account, the cabinet or council in exile can avoid inadvertently offending or alienating the target audience. Adapting strategies allows for the use of appropriate language, symbols, and cultural references that resonate with the local population.

3. Resource Optimization: Adapting strategies based on available resources is crucial for resource optimization. The cabinet or council in exile may have limited financial, human, or logistical resources. By understanding the available resources, they can plan and prioritize activities that are feasible and cost-effective. Adapting strategies helps them make the most of their resources and achieve maximum impact.

4. Flexibility and Agility: Adapting strategies allows the cabinet or council in exile to be flexible and agile in responding to changing circumstances. Political, social, and economic dynamics can evolve over time, requiring adjustments in their approach. By staying adaptable, they can seize opportunities, address emerging challenges, and respond to new developments in the target country. Flexibility and agility are key to maintaining relevance and effectiveness in their advocacy efforts.

5. Audience Engagement: Adapting strategies based on the target audience helps to enhance audience engagement. Different segments of the population may have varying levels of awareness, interests, and needs. By understanding the target audience's perspectives and concerns, the cabinet or council in exile can tailor their messages, activities, and channels of communication to effectively engage and mobilize support. This personalized approach helps to establish a connection and build trust with the audience.

6. Measuring Impact: Adapting strategies based on the specific context and target audience allows for better measurement of impact. By setting clear objectives and utilizing appropriate metrics, the cabinet or council in exile can assess the effectiveness of their strategies and make data-driven decisions. Measuring impact helps them identify what works and what doesn't, enabling them to refine their approach and optimize their efforts over time.

Overall, adapting strategies based on the specific context, target audience, and available resources is essential for the cabinet or council in exile to maximize their impact, ensure cultural sensitivity, optimize resources, stay flexible, engage the audience effectively, and measure their progress. It allows them to tailor their approach to the unique circumstances of the target country and increase their chances of success in raising awareness and garnering support for their cause.

Army and Hostile Revolutionary Sepa and Paramilitary forces:

When facing a hostile military faction loyal to an unpopular government, a cabinet in exile can take several steps and measures to address the situation. Here are some possible actions they can consider:

1. Diplomatic Outreach: The cabinet in exile should engage in diplomatic outreach to foreign governments, international organizations, and regional bodies. They can seek diplomatic recognition, support, and assistance in addressing the hostile military faction. This can involve diplomatic negotiations, lobbying, and advocacy to garner international pressure on the unpopular government and the military faction.

2. International Alliances: The cabinet in exile should seek to build alliances with other countries or organizations that have an interest in promoting democracy, human rights, or stability in the target country. By forming strategic partnerships, they can strengthen their position and gain support in addressing the hostile military faction. This can involve diplomatic negotiations, cooperation agreements, or joint initiatives.

3. Security and Defense: The cabinet in exile should assess their security situation and take measures to ensure the safety of their members, supporters, and assets. This can involve implementing security protocols, establishing secure communication channels, and seeking protection from international entities. They may also explore options for building a defense force or seeking military assistance from friendly countries or international peacekeeping forces.

4. Mobilizing Civil Society: The cabinet in exile should actively engage and mobilize civil society within the target country. They can work with local organizations, activists, and community leaders to build a broad-based movement against the unpopular government and the hostile military faction. This can involve organizing protests, strikes, and other forms of nonviolent resistance to put pressure on the military faction and raise awareness among the general population.

5. Information and Communication: The cabinet in exile should utilize various communication channels to disseminate information and counter propaganda from the unpopular government and the military faction. They can establish their own media outlets, use social media platforms, and collaborate with independent journalists to share their message, expose human rights abuses, and highlight the

illegitimacy of the military faction. Information campaigns can help to rally domestic and international support.

6. Humanitarian Assistance: The cabinet in exile should prioritize providing humanitarian assistance to the affected population within the target country. This can involve organizing relief efforts, coordinating with international humanitarian organizations, and addressing the immediate needs of vulnerable groups. By demonstrating their commitment to the well-being of the people, the cabinet in exile can gain credibility and support.
7. Legal and Accountability Measures: The cabinet in exile should work towards legal accountability for human rights abuses committed by the military faction. They can document evidence, work with international human rights organizations, and seek avenues for justice, such as international criminal tribunals or truth and reconciliation commissions. Pursuing legal measures can help delegitimize the military faction and build a case for international intervention.
8. International Sanctions: The cabinet in exile can advocate for targeted sanctions against individuals or entities associated with the hostile military faction. They can engage with foreign governments, international organizations, and civil society to impose diplomatic, economic, or travel restrictions on those responsible for human rights abuses or supporting the military faction. International sanctions can put pressure on the faction and isolate them from sources of support.
9. International Advocacy: The cabinet in exile can engage in international advocacy efforts to raise awareness about the situation and garner support from the international community. They can utilize diplomatic channels, international organizations, and media platforms to highlight the illegitimacy of the unpopular government and the actions of the hostile military faction. This can involve lobbying for sanctions, resolutions, or diplomatic pressure on the faction and the government.
10. Building Coalitions: The cabinet in exile can work towards building coalitions with domestic opposition groups, civil society organizations, and other stakeholders who are also opposed to the unpopular government and the military faction. By forming alliances, they can amplify their voice, strengthen their position, and coordinate efforts to challenge the faction's control. This can involve joint statements, collaborative actions, and shared strategies.
11. Mobilizing Public Support: The cabinet in exile can focus on mobilizing public support within the target country and internationally. They can engage in public campaigns, use social media platforms, and organize protests or demonstrations to raise awareness and rally support against the faction and the unpopular government. Mobilizing public sentiment can put pressure on the faction and create momentum for change.
12. Engaging with the Military: The cabinet in exile can explore opportunities for dialogue and engagement with members of the military who may be disenchanted

with the faction or sympathetic to the cause. This can involve reaching out to military leaders or individual soldiers, highlighting the negative consequences of their actions, and presenting an alternative vision for a more inclusive and democratic future. Engaging with the military can help weaken the faction's support base.

13. Establishing Shadow Governance: The cabinet in exile can establish a shadow governance structure that represents the legitimate interests and aspirations of the people. This can involve creating ministries or departments that address key areas such as education, health, and finance. By demonstrating effective governance and providing services to the population, the cabinet in exile can undermine the credibility of the unpopular government and the faction.

14. Legal and Accountability Measures: The cabinet in exile can pursue legal and accountability measures against the faction and the unpopular government. They can document human rights abuses, collect evidence of crimes, and work with international human rights organizations to seek justice through international courts or tribunals. Pursuing legal accountability can delegitimize the faction and provide a basis for international intervention or sanctions.

15. Support for Dissidents and Refugees: The cabinet in exile can provide support and protection for dissidents, activists, and refugees fleeing persecution from the faction and the unpopular government. This can involve setting up safe houses, providing legal assistance, and advocating for their rights and safety at the international level. Supporting dissidents and refugees can strengthen the opposition against the faction and expose their abuses.

16. International Humanitarian Assistance: The cabinet in exile can prioritize providing humanitarian assistance to the affected population within the target country. This can involve coordinating with international humanitarian organizations, organizing relief efforts, and addressing the immediate needs of vulnerable groups. By demonstrating their commitment to the well-being of the people, the cabinet in exile can gain credibility and support.

It is important for the cabinet in exile to assess the specific context, consult with experts, and carefully plan their actions to address the hostile military faction. They should also seek legal advice and consider the potential risks and consequences of their interventions. Collaboration with international partners, civil society, and the affected population is crucial for building a strong and unified front against the military faction and the unpopular government.

Peace and stability:

To establish peace and a functioning cabinet in exile as a temporary government, the following steps can be taken:

1. Negotiate a Peaceful Transition: Engage in negotiations with all relevant parties, including the former government and any opposition factions, to ensure a peaceful transition of power. Establish a framework for dialogue and mediation to address

grievances and build consensus on the way forward.

2. Form a Transitional Cabinet: Assemble a diverse and inclusive transitional cabinet that represents different sectors of society, including political parties, civil society organizations, and ethnic or religious groups. This will help ensure broad representation and inclusivity in decision-making processes.
3. Develop a Transitional Constitution: Draft a transitional constitution that outlines the principles, values, and mechanisms for governance during the transitional period. This constitution should emphasize democratic principles, human rights, and the rule of law, while also addressing the specific challenges and needs of the country.
4. Implement Transitional Justice Measures: Institute transitional justice mechanisms to address past human rights abuses, promote reconciliation, and provide justice for victims. This may include truth and reconciliation commissions, reparations programs, and legal proceedings for perpetrators of gross violations.
5. Restore Basic Services and Infrastructure: Prioritize the restoration of basic services, such as healthcare, education, water, and electricity, to ensure the well-being of the population. Invest in rebuilding infrastructure that may have been damaged during the conflict, focusing on areas with the greatest need.
6. Ensure Security and Rule of Law: Establish security forces that are accountable, professional, and representative of the diversity of the population. Strengthen the rule of law by reforming the judicial system, enhancing legal protections, and promoting respect for human rights.
7. Engage in Economic Recovery: Develop a comprehensive economic recovery plan that addresses the country's immediate needs and sets the foundation for sustainable development. This may involve attracting foreign investment, promoting entrepreneurship, and providing support for small and medium-sized enterprises.
8. Foster International Support: Seek international support and cooperation to aid in the transitional process. Engage with regional organizations, international donors, and other stakeholders to secure financial assistance, technical expertise, and diplomatic support.
9. Communicate with the Population: Maintain open and transparent communication with the population to build trust and foster a sense of ownership in the transitional process. Utilize various communication channels, such as town hall meetings, public consultations, and media platforms, to ensure that the concerns and aspirations of the people are heard and addressed.
10. Plan for Elections and Democratic Transition: Develop a roadmap for democratic elections and a smooth transition to a permanent government. This should include establishing an independent electoral commission, implementing voter education programs, and ensuring a level playing field for all political parties.

It is important to note that the specific steps may vary depending on the context and challenges faced by each country. Flexibility, inclusivity, and a commitment to the principles of democracy, human rights, and rule of law are crucial in establishing a peaceful and functioning cabinet in exile as a temporary government.

Transition and Country Representation:

A transitional cabinet can ensure broad representation and inclusivity in decision-making processes through the following measures:

1. Inclusive Selection Process: The transitional cabinet should be formed through an inclusive and transparent selection process. This process should involve consultations with various stakeholders, including political parties, civil society organizations, ethnic and religious groups, and marginalized communities. It should aim to include individuals who have diverse backgrounds, expertise, and perspectives.

2. Gender and Minority Representation: Pay special attention to gender and minority representation in the transitional cabinet. Actively seek the participation of women and individuals from marginalized communities to ensure their voices are heard and their needs are addressed. This can be achieved through targeted outreach, quotas, or affirmative action measures.

3. Regional and Ethnic Balance: Strive for regional and ethnic balance in the composition of the transitional cabinet. This will help ensure that different regions and ethnic groups are adequately represented and have a say in decision-making processes. Consider the demographic realities and historical grievances of the country when determining the representation.

4. Expertise and Competence: Select individuals for the transitional cabinet based on their expertise, competence, and experience in relevant fields. This will help ensure that the cabinet has the necessary skills and knowledge to address the challenges faced by the country during the transitional period.

5. Consultative Approach: Adopt a consultative approach in decision-making processes. Engage with a wide range of stakeholders, including civil society organizations, community leaders, and experts, to gather diverse perspectives and inputs. This can be done through regular meetings, public consultations, and advisory committees.

6. Transparency and Accountability: Maintain transparency in the decision-making processes of the transitional cabinet. Communicate the rationale behind decisions and provide opportunities for public scrutiny and feedback. Establish mechanisms for accountability to ensure that the cabinet members are held responsible for their actions.

7. Outreach and Engagement: Actively engage with the population through various means of communication. Use media platforms, town hall meetings, and online platforms to disseminate information, gather feedback, and involve the public in decision-making processes. Encourage public participation and involvement in shaping policies and programs.
8. Capacity Building: Invest in capacity building programs to enhance the skills and knowledge of cabinet members. Provide training and support to help them effectively carry out their responsibilities and make informed decisions. This will contribute to the effectiveness and inclusivity of the transitional cabinet.
9. Regular Evaluation and Feedback: Establish mechanisms for regular evaluation and feedback on the performance of the transitional cabinet. Solicit feedback from different stakeholders, including the public, to assess the effectiveness of decision-making processes and identify areas for improvement.

By implementing these measures, a transitional cabinet can ensure broader representation and inclusivity in decision-making processes, leading to more effective and legitimate governance during the transitional period.

Regional and Ethnic Balance:

Regional and ethnic balance plays a crucial role in ensuring broad representation and inclusivity in decision-making processes for several reasons:

1. Representation of Diverse Perspectives: Regional and ethnic balance in the composition of decision-making bodies helps ensure that the diverse perspectives and interests of different regions and ethnic groups are adequately represented. It allows for a more comprehensive understanding of the needs, priorities, and challenges faced by various communities within the country.
2. Overcoming Marginalization: In many countries, certain regions or ethnic groups have historically been marginalized or excluded from political processes. By prioritizing regional and ethnic balance, decision-making bodies can address historical inequalities and provide a platform for marginalized communities to have a voice in shaping policies and programs.
3. Building Trust and Social Cohesion: In societies with ethnic or regional divisions, ensuring regional and ethnic balance in decision-making processes can help build trust and promote social cohesion. It sends a powerful message that all communities are valued and have an equal stake in the governance of the country. This can contribute to a sense of belonging and unity among different groups, reducing tensions and promoting stability.
4. Conflict Prevention and Resolution: Regional and ethnic imbalances in decision-making can be a source of social and political unrest. By promoting regional and

ethnic balance, decision-making bodies can help prevent conflicts or mitigate existing tensions. It demonstrates a commitment to addressing grievances and resolving disputes through inclusive and participatory processes.

5. Effective Policy Implementation: Policies and programs that are developed with input from diverse regions and ethnic groups are more likely to be effective and sustainable. Decision-making bodies that include representatives from different backgrounds can draw upon a wider range of experiences, knowledge, and expertise, leading to more informed and contextually relevant decisions.
6. Legitimacy and Public Trust: A decision-making body that reflects the regional and ethnic diversity of a country is more likely to be seen as legitimate and representative by the population. This enhances public trust in the decision-making process and increases the likelihood of acceptance and support for the decisions made.
7. It is important to note that regional and ethnic balance should not be seen as a tokenistic gesture, but rather as a genuine commitment to inclusivity and equal representation. It should be accompanied by efforts to ensure meaningful participation, equal access to resources and opportunities, and the empowerment of all communities within the country.

Rebuilding Iran Healthcare Systems

Morality and Self-worth

Rebuilding morality in healthcare workers who have been mistreated and professionally abused in a corrupt system is a complex and challenging process. It requires a comprehensive approach that addresses both the individual and systemic factors contributing to the mistreatment. Here are some steps that can help in rebuilding morality:

1. Acknowledge and Validate: Recognize and acknowledge the mistreatment and professional abuse experienced by healthcare workers. Validate their feelings, emotions, and the impact it has had on their well-being. Create a safe and supportive environment where they can openly express their experiences and concerns.

2. Provide Support and Counseling: Offer psychological support and counseling services to healthcare workers who have been mistreated. This can help them process their emotions, trauma, and build resilience. Encourage them to seek professional help and provide access to resources for mental health support.

3. Foster a Culture of Respect and Dignity: Take proactive steps to foster a culture of respect, dignity, and psychological safety within the healthcare institution. Develop and enforce policies that prohibit mistreatment and abuse. Provide training and education on professional ethics, communication skills, and conflict resolution to all healthcare staff.

4. Encourage Open Communication: Promote open and transparent communication channels where healthcare workers can freely express their concerns, ideas, and suggestions. Encourage reporting of mistreatment and provide multiple avenues for reporting, such as anonymous reporting systems, to protect those who fear retaliation.

5. Establish Support Networks: Create support networks or peer support programs where healthcare workers can connect with and seek support from their colleagues who have experienced similar mistreatment. These networks can provide a safe space for sharing experiences, seeking advice, and finding solidarity.

6. Address Systemic Issues: Identify and address the systemic issues contributing to the mistreatment and professional abuse. This may involve conducting thorough investigations, holding individuals accountable for their actions, and implementing structural changes to prevent future mistreatment. Involve healthcare workers in the decision-making processes to ensure their voices are heard.

7. Provide Training and Education: Offer ongoing training and education programs on professional ethics, moral decision-making, and compassionate care. Equip healthcare workers with the knowledge and skills necessary to navigate ethical dilemmas and make morally sound decisions in challenging situations.

8. Promote Work-Life Balance: Recognize the importance of work-life balance and support healthcare workers in maintaining their physical and mental well-being. Implement policies that prioritize self-care, minimize burnout, and create a healthy work environment.

9. Cultivate Leadership and Role Models: Foster leadership that embodies and promotes ethical behavior, empathy, and compassion. Cultivate role models within the healthcare institution who can inspire and guide healthcare workers in rebuilding their morality.

10. Advocate for Change: Encourage healthcare workers to engage in advocacy efforts that aim to address systemic issues and promote positive change in the healthcare system. Support initiatives that advocate for fair treatment, ethical practices, and patient-centered care.

11. Addressing Trauma: Professional mistreatment and abuse can have long-lasting effects on the mental and emotional well-being of healthcare workers. It is important to recognize and address the trauma they have experienced. Trauma-informed care and support services should be provided to help them heal and recover.

12. Ethical Decision-Making: Healthcare workers may have been forced to compromise their ethical principles due to the corrupt system they were in. Providing training and education on ethical decision-making can help them regain confidence in their ability to make morally sound choices in their practice.

13. Building Trust: Rebuilding trust among healthcare workers is crucial. Trust in the healthcare system and its leaders may have been eroded due to the mistreatment and abuse they have faced. Transparency, accountability, and consistent actions that prioritize the well-being of healthcare workers are essential in rebuilding trust.

14. Advocacy and Policy Change: Healthcare workers who have experienced mistreatment can play a crucial role in advocating for policy changes and reforms within the healthcare system. Encouraging them to speak out and share their experiences can bring attention to the need for systemic change and hold those responsible accountable.

15. Encouraging Empathy and Compassion: Promoting empathy and compassion in healthcare workers is essential to rebuilding morality. Encourage them to reflect on their experiences and the impact it has had on their own well-being, as well as the well-being of their patients. Cultivating empathy can help healthcare workers reconnect with their intrinsic motivation to provide compassionate care.

16. Supportive Leadership: Strong and supportive leadership is crucial in rebuilding morality. Leaders should actively listen to the concerns and experiences of healthcare workers, provide guidance and support, and hold individuals accountable for their actions. Leaders should also model ethical behavior and create an environment that encourages open communication and respect.

17. Continuous Evaluation and Improvement: Regularly evaluate the effectiveness of the implemented changes and interventions. Seek feedback from healthcare workers and adjust

as needed. Continuous improvement is essential to ensure that the rebuilding process is effective and sustainable.

It is important to note that rebuilding morality in healthcare workers is a long-term process that requires commitment and collaboration from all stakeholders involved. It involves addressing individual needs, systemic issues, and creating a culture that values ethics, respect, and compassion. By taking these steps, we can work towards rebuilding the moral foundation of healthcare and promoting a healthier and more ethical healthcare system for both healthcare workers and patients.

Rebuilding morality in healthcare workers requires a collective effort from healthcare institutions, leaders, and individuals. It is important to create an environment that values and upholds ethical standards, supports those who have been mistreated, and works towards preventing future abuse.

Professional Trauma and Morality Damage:

Trauma-informed care and support services can provide significant help to healthcare workers who have experienced mistreatment and abuse. Here are some ways in which trauma-informed care can be beneficial:

1. Validation and Empowerment: Trauma-informed care acknowledges the experiences and feelings of healthcare workers who have been mistreated and abused. It validates their emotions and empowers them to recognize that their reactions are normal responses to abnormal situations. This validation can help alleviate feelings of self-blame or shame.

2. Safety and Trust: Trauma-informed care creates a safe and supportive environment for healthcare workers. It prioritizes physical and emotional safety, ensuring that individuals feel secure and protected. This can help rebuild trust in the healthcare system and those providing support.

3. Trauma Education: Healthcare workers who have experienced mistreatment may not fully understand the impact of trauma on their mental and emotional well-being. Trauma-informed care provides education and information about trauma, its effects, and coping strategies. This knowledge can help healthcare workers make sense of their experiences and develop effective self-care strategies.

4. Emotional Regulation: Trauma-informed care teaches healthcare workers techniques to regulate their emotions and manage stress. This may include mindfulness exercises, breathing techniques, or other relaxation methods. Learning these skills can help healthcare workers cope with the psychological distress caused by mistreatment and abuse.

5. Trauma-Focused Therapy: Trauma-informed care may involve individual or group therapy sessions that specifically address the trauma experienced by healthcare workers. Trauma-focused therapies, such as cognitive-behavioral therapy (CBT) or eye movement desensitization and reprocessing (EMDR), can help individuals process their traumatic

experiences, reduce distressing symptoms, and promote healing.

6. Self-Care and Resilience Building: Trauma-informed care emphasizes the importance of self-care and resilience-building activities. Healthcare workers are encouraged to engage in activities that promote their well-being, such as exercise, hobbies, social support, and self-reflection. Building resilience can help healthcare workers bounce back from adversity and maintain their mental and emotional well-being.

7. Peer Support: Trauma-informed care often includes peer support groups where healthcare workers can connect with others who have had similar experiences. Peer support provides a sense of belonging, validation, and understanding. Sharing experiences and supporting each other can be incredibly healing and can help reduce feelings of isolation.

Trauma-informed care and support services can provide significant help to healthcare workers who have experienced mistreatment and abuse. Here are some ways in which trauma-informed care can be beneficial:

By implementing trauma-informed care and support services, healthcare workers who have experienced mistreatment and abuse can receive the understanding, validation, and resources they need to heal and recover. It helps them develop healthy coping mechanisms, regain a sense of control, and restore their overall well-being.

Trauma-informed care prioritizes physical and emotional safety for healthcare workers by implementing the following strategies:

1. Creating a Safe Environment: Trauma-informed care ensures that the physical environment is safe and secure. This may involve measures such as well-lit spaces, clear pathways, and secure entrances. It also includes implementing policies and procedures to prevent mistreatment and abuse within healthcare settings.

2. Establishing Trust and Transparency: Trauma-informed care emphasizes the importance of building trusting relationships between healthcare workers and their supervisors, colleagues, and support staff. This involves open and transparent communication, active listening, and respect for boundaries. Trust is crucial for healthcare workers to feel safe and secure in their work environment.

3. Trauma-Informed Policies and Procedures: Trauma-informed care involves the development and implementation of policies and procedures that consider the impact of trauma on healthcare workers. These policies aim to prevent re-traumatization and ensure that individuals are not exposed to further harm. For example, policies may address issues such as workplace bullying, harassment, and violence.

4. Trauma-Sensitive Language: Trauma-informed care recognizes the importance of using trauma-sensitive language when communicating with healthcare workers. This involves being mindful of the words used, avoiding blaming or shaming language, and using compassionate and supportive language instead. Trauma-sensitive language helps create a

safe and non-judgmental space for healthcare workers to share their experiences and seek support.

5. Emotional Support and Validation: Trauma-informed care provides healthcare workers with emotional support and validation for their experiences. This involves acknowledging and validating their emotions, feelings, and reactions to mistreatment and abuse. Healthcare workers are encouraged to express their emotions in a safe and supportive environment without fear of judgment or retribution.

6. Training and Education: Trauma-informed care includes training and education for healthcare workers and staff on trauma, its effects, and how to respond appropriately. This training helps create awareness and understanding of trauma and equips healthcare workers with the knowledge and skills to provide safe and supportive care to their colleagues.

7. Self-Care and Stress Management: Trauma-informed care emphasizes the importance of self-care and stress management for healthcare workers. It encourages individuals to prioritize their physical and emotional well-being through activities such as exercise, mindfulness, relaxation techniques, and seeking support from their support network.

By prioritizing physical and emotional safety through these strategies, trauma-informed care creates an environment where healthcare workers feel protected, supported, and able to heal from their traumatic experiences. It helps to prevent further harm and promotes the overall well-being of healthcare workers.

The role of trauma-sensitive language in trauma-informed care is to create a safe and supportive environment for individuals who have experienced trauma. It recognizes that the language we use can have a profound impact on how individuals perceive andrespond to their experiences. Trauma-sensitive language aims to minimize re-traumatization, promote healing, and foster a sense of safety and trust.

Here are some key aspects of trauma-sensitive language:

1. Non-Blaming and Non-Shaming: Trauma-sensitive language avoids blaming or shaming individuals for their experiences. It recognizes that trauma is not the fault of the person who experienced it and avoids language that implies otherwise. Instead, it focuses on understanding and empathy.

2. Empowering and Strength-Based: Trauma-sensitive language acknowledges the resilience and strength of individuals who have experienced trauma. It emphasizes their ability to heal and recover, rather than defining them solely by their traumatic experiences. It promotes a sense of empowerment and instills hope.

3. Compassionate and Supportive: Trauma-sensitive language is compassionate and supportive. It acknowledges the pain and suffering that trauma can cause and expresses empathy and understanding. It creates a safe space for individuals to share their experiences and seek support without fear of judgment or stigma.

4. Clear and Respectful: Trauma-sensitive language is clear and respectful in its

communication. It avoids using jargon, ambiguous terms, or offensive language. It respects the individual's boundaries and preferences for discussing their trauma.

5. Mindful of Triggers: Trauma-sensitive language is mindful of potential triggers that may re-activate traumatic memories or emotions. It avoids using language or discussing topics that may be distressing or triggering for the individual. This includes being cautious about graphic details or graphic imagery.

6. Inclusive and Culturally Sensitive: Trauma-sensitive language is inclusive and culturally sensitive. It recognizes that different cultures may have different ways of understanding and expressing trauma. It respects and honors cultural beliefs, practices, and language preferences.

Furthermore, trauma sensitive language includes and support:

1. Person-Centered: Trauma-sensitive language focuses on the person, their experiences, and their needs. It recognizes that everyone's experience of trauma is unique and respects their autonomy and agency in sharing their story.

2. Validation and Empathy: Trauma-sensitive language acknowledges and validates the emotions, thoughts, and reactions of individuals who have experienced trauma. It expresses empathy and understanding, letting them know that their experiences are valid and that they are not alone.

3. Non-Judgmental: Trauma-sensitive language avoids judgment or assumptions about the individual or their experiences. It recognizes that trauma is not the fault of the person who experienced it and refrains from blaming or shaming language.

4. Safety and Boundaries: Trauma-sensitive language creates a safe space for individuals to share their experiences or thoughts. It respects their boundaries and allows them to disclose as much or as little as they are comfortable with. It also ensures that conversations around trauma are conducted in a confidential and secure manner.

5. Clarity and Simplicity: Trauma-sensitive language uses clear and simple language to avoid confusion or misunderstanding. It avoids using complex or technical terms that may be overwhelming or triggering for the individual.

6. Trauma-Informed: Trauma-sensitive language incorporates an understanding of trauma's impact on individuals and their responses. It considers the potential triggers and avoids language or topics that may retraumatize or cause distress.

7. Culturally Sensitive: Trauma-sensitive language recognizes and respects cultural differences in understanding and expressing trauma. It considers cultural beliefs, norms, and values, ensuring that communication is culturally sensitive and inclusive.

8. Establishing Trust: Using trauma-sensitive language helps build trust between the speaker and the listener. It communicates empathy, understanding, and acceptance, which are essential for individuals who have experienced trauma to feel safe and comfortable sharing their experiences.

9. Validation and Empathy: Trauma-sensitive language acknowledges and validates the emotions, thoughts, and reactions of individuals who have experienced trauma. It expresses empathy and understanding, letting them know that their experiences are valid and that they are not alone. This validation helps create a safe environment where they feel heard and understood.

10. Non-Judgmental Attitude: Trauma-sensitive language avoids judgment or assumptions about the individual or their experiences. It recognizes that trauma is not the fault of the person who experienced it and refrains from blaming or shaming language. By creating a non-judgmental atmosphere, individuals feel more comfortable sharing their experiences without fear of being criticized or stigmatized.

11. Respecting Boundaries: Trauma-sensitive language respects the boundaries of individuals who have experienced trauma. It allows them to disclose as much or as little as they are comfortable with. By honoring their boundaries, individuals feel a sense of control over their narrative and can share at a pace that feels safe for them.

12. Confidentiality: Trauma-sensitive language ensures that conversations around trauma are conducted in a confidential and secure manner. This confidentiality helps individuals feel reassured that their experiences will be treated with respect and privacy, further enhancing their sense of safety.

13.Trauma-Informed Approach: Trauma-sensitive language incorporates an understanding of trauma's impact on individuals and their responses. It avoids language or topics that may retraumatize or cause distress. By being trauma-informed, individuals feel protected from potential triggers, allowing them to share their experiences without fear of traumatization.

14.Active Listening: Trauma-sensitive language involves active listening, where the listener is fully present and attentive to the speaker's needs. It involves providing space for the individual to express themselves and validating their emotions. Active listening helps individuals feel heard, valued, and supported, contributing to the creation of a safe space for sharing.

By incorporating these aspects into our language and interactions, we can create a supportive and understanding environment for individuals who have experienced trauma, facilitating their healing and recovery.

By using trauma-sensitive language, healthcare providers, therapists, and other professionals can create a safe and supportive environment for individuals who have experienced trauma. It helps to build trust, promote healing, and empower individuals on their journey towards recovery.

The benefits of using trauma-sensitive language in creating a safe space for individuals to share their experiences include:

1. Increased Trust: Trauma-sensitive language helps build trust between the speaker and the listener. When individuals feel that their experiences are acknowledged and understood,

they are more likely to trust the person they are sharing with. This trust creates a safe environment where they can openly express themselves without fear of judgment or rejection.

2. Enhanced Emotional Safety: Trauma-sensitive language creates an emotionally safe space for individuals to share their experiences. It communicates empathy, validation, and acceptance, which are crucial for individuals who have experienced trauma. Feeling emotionally safe encourages them to open up and share their experiences more freely.

3. Validation and Empowerment: Trauma-sensitive language validates the experiences, emotions, and reactions of individuals who have experienced trauma. It acknowledges their pain, courage, and resilience, letting them know that their experiences are valid and that they are not alone. This validation empowers individuals to share their stories and helps them feel heard and understood.

4. Reduced Stigma and Shame: Trauma-sensitive language avoids blaming or shaming individuals for their experiences. It recognizes that trauma is not the fault of the person who experienced it and refrains from using language that perpetuates stigma or judgment. By eliminating shame and stigma, individuals feel more comfortable sharing their experiences without fear of being stigmatized or blamed.

5. Increased Sense of Control: Trauma-sensitive language respects the boundaries and autonomy of individuals who have experienced trauma. It allows them to disclose as much or as little as they are comfortable with, giving them a sense of control over their narrative. This increased sense of control enables individuals to share their experiences at their own pace and in a way that feels safe for them.

6. Building a Supportive Community: Using trauma-sensitive language fosters a supportive community where individuals feel understood and accepted. It creates an environment where people can empathize with each other's experiences, provide support, and learn from one another. This sense of community promotes healing, resilience, and a stronger support network.

7. Trauma-Informed Care: Trauma-sensitive language is a crucial aspect of trauma-informed care. By using language that is informed by an understanding of trauma's impact, individuals feel safer and more supported. Trauma-informed care acknowledges the potential triggers and sensitivities associated with trauma and avoids traumatization, promoting a safe space for sharing.

Validation is important when using trauma-sensitive language with individuals who have experienced trauma because it acknowledges and affirms their experiences, emotions, and reactions. Here are some reasons why validation is crucial:

1. Affirmation of Reality: Trauma can often lead to feelings of confusion, self-doubt, and disbelief. By validating their experiences, individuals are reassured that what they went through was real and valid. It helps them regain a sense of certainty and clarity about their own experiences, reducing self-blame and self-doubt.

2. Emotional Support: Validation provides emotional support to individuals who have experienced trauma. It communicates empathy, understanding, and acceptance, which can be incredibly comforting. Knowing that their feelings and reactions are acknowledged and accepted can help individuals feel less alone, understood, and supported.

3. Normalization of Reactions: Trauma can elicit a wide range of emotional and physical responses, which may sometimes feel overwhelming or irrational. Validating these reactions helps individuals understand that their responses are normal and understandable given their traumatic experiences. It helps them recognize that their reactions are not their fault and that others have had similar experiences.

4. Rebuilding Trust: Trauma can often erode trust in oneself and others. Validation helps rebuild trust by demonstrating that their experiences and feelings are taken seriously and respected. It shows that the person using trauma-sensitive language is a safe and trustworthy individual who can be relied upon for support and understanding.

5. Empowerment and Agency: Validation empowers individuals by affirming their autonomy and agency. It recognizes that they have the right to their feelings, thoughts, and experiences and that they are the experts of their own lives. This empowerment can help individuals regain a sense of control and confidence in themselves and their ability to navigate their healing journey.

6. Counteracting Stigma and Shame: Trauma can often be associated with stigma and shame, leading individuals to feel isolated and judged. Validation helps counteract these negative feelings by communicating that their experiences are not their fault and that they are not alone. It helps reduce self-blame and encourages individuals to seek support and healing without fear of judgment or rejection.

7. Building Therapeutic Alliance: Validation is a fundamental aspect of building a strong therapeutic alliance. When individuals feel validated, they are more likely to trust and connect with their therapists or support systems. This alliance is essential for effective therapy and support, as it provides a safe and supportive space for individuals to explore their trauma and work towards healing.

Overall, trauma-sensitive language plays a vital role in creating a safe space for individuals to share their experiences. It builds trust, validates emotions, reduces stigma, and empowers individuals to share their stories. By using trauma-sensitive language, we can foster a supportive and healing environment for those who have experienced trauma.

In summary, morality validation is crucial when using trauma-sensitive language because it affirms the reality of individuals' experiences, provides emotional support, normalizes reactions, rebuilds trust, empowers individuals, counteracts stigma and shame, and strengthens the therapeutic alliance. It is an essential component of creating a safe and supportive environment for individuals who have experienced trauma.

Rebuilding Iran: Evolving democracy

Introduction

This narrative addresses the pressing issue of fighting tyranny and dictatorship and proposes a plan of action for a peaceful transition towards democracy, freedom, and a secular country. Such change requires a well-organized strategy and a clear manifesto to guide us in our efforts.

The first stage in this process is raising awareness and mobilizing the population. It is crucial to educate the public about the harms of tyranny and dictatorship and to foster a collective understanding of the benefits of democracy, freedom, and secularism. This can be achieved through various means such as public campaigns, educational programs, and grassroots movements.

The second stage involves building a united front against the oppressive regime. This requires the collaboration and cooperation of various sectors of society, including political parties, civil society organizations, human rights activists, and religious leaders who advocate for tolerance and inclusivity. By uniting diverse voices, we can present a strong and unified front against tyranny and dictatorship.

The third stage focuses on peaceful resistance and nonviolent forms of protest. This includes organizing peaceful demonstrations, strikes, and other acts of civil disobedience to put pressure on the regime and demand change. It is important to emphasize the power of nonviolence and the need to protect human rights during these actions.

The fourth stage entails international engagement and support. It is crucial to garner international attention and support for the cause of democracy and freedom. This can be achieved through diplomatic efforts, lobbying, and engaging with international organizations and human rights bodies. International solidarity can provide additional leverage and create pressure on the oppressive regime to enact change.

The final stage involves a carefully planned transition to democracy. This includes drafting a constitution that upholds democratic principles, ensuring free and fair elections, and establishing institutions that safeguard human rights and the rule of law. It is essential to involve all segments of society in this process to ensure inclusivity and prevent the rise of new forms of oppression.

In conclusion, fighting tyranny and dictatorship requires a well-coordinated plan of action and a clear manifesto. By following these stages, we can work towards a peaceful transition to a democratic, free, and secular country. We must stand against tyranny and advocate for the values that promote human dignity, freedom, and justice.

Subversive Manifesto:

The proposed manifesto outlines multiple stages for the transition in Iran. Here are some of the key stages:

1. Forming an effective and politically savvy replacement government in exile: This stage involves establishing a government in exile that can effectively represent the interests of the Iranian people and garner international support.
2. Creating a bridge between the government in exile and activists in Iran: Communication and coordination between the government in exile and activists within Iran are crucial to support their efforts for change.
3. Disseminating information and propaganda exposing Islamic crimes: Volunteers both inside and outside Iran can be mobilized to disseminate information and expose the human rights violations committed by the current regime.
4. Forming alliances with Western democracies and gaining recognition: Building alliances with democratic countries and gaining international recognition for the government in exile will strengthen its legitimacy and support.
5. Establishing working relationships with military factions open to reconciliation: Identifying military factions that are open-minded to reconciliation and support for a secular democracy is important for a smooth transition. Working with these factions can help establish the rule of law and ensure security nationwide.
6. Forming a group of technocrats and scholars to support government affairs: A team of technocrats and scholars can be formed to provide expertise and support in various areas, ensuring the smooth functioning of the government.
7. Creating a portfolio to maintain emergency services and healthcare systems: A portfolio dedicated to maintaining emergency services and healthcare systems will ensure the well-being of the population during the transition period.
8. Attracting foreign investors and international workers: Attracting foreign investment, international workers, and financial institutions will help create a thriving economy and boost the country's development.
9. Reorganizing the military and Sepah: Bringing the military and Sepah (Islamic Revolutionary Guard Corps) under one system will streamline and strengthen the security forces.
10. Announcing national reconciliation and sanctuary: Declaring national reconciliation and offering sanctuary to all military personnel will promote unity and encourage support for the new government.
11. Reorganizing the justice department: Restructuring the justice department will ensure a fair and impartial legal system based on human rights and freedom.

12. Detaining those involved in crimes: Holding accountable those involved in torture, abuse, mass murder, and unjust killings will promote justice and provide closure to the victims and their families.

These stages highlight some of the key steps outlined in the proposed manifest for the transition in Iran. Each stage requires careful planning, coordination, and international support to ensure a successful transition to a secular democratic government.

Forming Alliances:

1. Legitimacy: Gaining recognition from democratic countries lends legitimacy to the government in exile and its mission to establish a secular democratic government in Iran. It demonstrates that the international community acknowledges and supports the aspirations of the Iranian people for freedom, human rights, and democracy.
2. Political Support: Western democracies can provide political support to the government in exile by advocating for its cause, raising awareness about the human rights abuses in Iran, and putting pressure on the current regime to initiate democratic reforms. This support can help strengthen the position of the government in exile and its ability to mobilize international efforts for change.
3. Economic Assistance: Western democracies can provide economic assistance, including foreign aid, investment, and technical expertise, to support the transition process and the development of a new government in Iran. This assistance can help stabilize the economy, create jobs, and improve the living conditions of the Iranian people.
4. Security Cooperation: Building alliances with Western democracies can facilitate security cooperation, including intelligence sharing, training, and capacity-building for the military and security forces of the new government. This collaboration can help establish and maintain stability, counter extremist threats, and ensure the security of the Iranian people during the transition period.
5. Access to Resources and Technology: Western democracies can provide access to resources, technology, and best practices in various sectors such as healthcare, education, infrastructure, and governance. This exchange of knowledge and expertise can contribute to the development and modernization of Iran's institutions and systems.
6. International Pressure: By forming alliances with Western democracies, the government in exile can mobilize international pressure on the current regime to respect human rights, release political prisoners, and initiate democratic reforms. This pressure can increase the chances of a peaceful transition and discourage the regime from resorting to violence or repression.
7. Overall, forming alliances with Western democracies and gaining international recognition is crucial for the success of the transition in Iran. It provides the government in exile with political, economic, and security support, while also increasing the chances of international intervention and pressure to facilitate a peaceful and democratic change in the country.

International Coalition:

1. Foreign Aid: Western democracies can provide financial support in the form of foreign aid to help fund the transition process. This aid can be used to address immediate humanitarian needs, support infrastructure development, and stimulate economic growth.
2. Investment: Western democracies can encourage and facilitate foreign direct investment (FDI) in Iran. This investment can help create jobs, boost economic development, and attract international businesses to contribute to the country's growth.
3. Technical Expertise: Western democracies can share technical expertise and best practices in various sectors such as governance, healthcare, education, agriculture, and infrastructure. This knowledge transfer can assist in building institutional capacity and improving the efficiency and effectiveness of government services.
4. Trade Agreements: Western democracies can negotiate trade agreements with the new government in Iran, facilitating increased trade and market access. These agreements can help diversify Iran's economy, promote exports, and attract foreign investment.
5. Financial Institutions: Western democracies can support the establishment or restructuring of financial institutions in Iran, such as banks, to ensure a stable financial system. This support can include technical assistance, training, and regulatory frameworks to promote transparency and accountability.
6. Development Programs: Western democracies can implement development programs that focus on poverty alleviation, job creation, and social welfare. These programs can help address the socio-economic challenges faced by the Iranian population and contribute to a more inclusive and equitable society.
7. Entrepreneurship and Small Business Support: Western democracies can provide support for entrepreneurship and small business development in Iran. This can include training programs, access to capital, mentoring, and networking opportunities, which can foster innovation, create employment opportunities, and drive economic growth.
8. Technology Transfer: Western democracies can facilitate the transfer of advanced technologies to Iran, particularly in sectors such as renewable energy, information technology, and manufacturing. This transfer can help modernize industries, improve productivity, and promote sustainable development.
9. Debt Relief or Restructuring: Western democracies can work with international financial institutions to provide debt relief or restructuring options for Iran. This can alleviate the burden of external debt and free up resources for investment in infrastructure, social programs, and economic development.
10. By offering economic assistance in these various forms, western democracies can play a significant role in supporting the transition process in Iran and contributing to the country's long-term stability, prosperity, and democratic development.

Western Democracy role:

1. Infrastructure Development: Western democracies can assist in the development of critical infrastructure such as transportation networks, energy systems, water supply, and telecommunications. This support can help modernize and expand infrastructure networks, improve connectivity, and enhance the overall economic development of Iran.

2. Energy and Renewable Resources: Western democracies can provide expertise and investment in the energy sector, including the development of renewable energy resources such as solar, wind, and hydroelectric power. This support can help diversify Iran's energy sources, reduce reliance on fossil fuels, and promote sustainable development.

3. Agriculture and Food Security: Western democracies can offer agricultural expertise, technology, and investment to enhance productivity, improve agricultural practices, and promote food security. This support can help modernize farming techniques, increase crop yields, and ensure a stable food supply for the Iranian population.

4. Healthcare and Pharmaceuticals: Western democracies can contribute to the improvement of healthcare infrastructure, training of healthcare professionals, and provision of medical equipment and supplies. They can also assist in the development of pharmaceutical industries, research, and access to affordable and quality healthcare services.

5. Education and Skill Development: Western democracies can support the enhancement of the education system by providing technical assistance, teacher training, curriculum development, and access to educational resources. They can also facilitate student exchanges and scholarships to promote academic and cultural exchange between Iran and Western countries.

6. Financial Services and Banking: Western democracies can assist in the development and modernization of Iran's financial sector, including banking systems, regulatory frameworks, and financial institutions. This support can help promote transparency, accountability, and access to financial services for businesses and individuals.

7. Information Technology and Digital Economy: Western democracies can contribute to the development of Iran's digital economy by sharing expertise in areas such as cybersecurity, e-commerce, digital infrastructure, and innovation. This support can foster technological advancements, job creation, and economic growth in the digital sector.

8. Environmental Protection and Conservation: Western democracies can collaborate with Iran in environmental protection efforts, including the preservation of natural resources, biodiversity, and sustainable management of ecosystems. This support

can promote environmental sustainability and address climate change challenges.

9. Governance and Public Administration: Western democracies can offer expertise and technical assistance in strengthening governance structures, promoting transparency, accountability, and the rule of law. This support can help build effective and responsive institutions, enhance public administration, and promote good governance practices.

By aiding in these sectors, western democracies can contribute to the overall development and stability of Iran during the transition process, fostering economic growth, social progress, and sustainable development.

Oppositions and Diaspora:

1. Technical Expertise and Training: Western democracies can provide technical expertise and training to healthcare professionals in Iran. This can include specialized training programs, workshops, and exchanges that focus on improving clinical skills, healthcare management, and the implementation of best practices.
2. Infrastructure Development: Western democracies can assist in the development and modernization of healthcare infrastructure in Iran. This can involve providing financial support, technical assistance, and expertise in designing and constructing healthcare facilities, hospitals, clinics, and laboratories.
3. Medical Equipment and Supplies: Western democracies can contribute to the provision of essential medical equipment, supplies, and technologies. This can include donating or subsidizing the purchase of equipment such as diagnostic tools, imaging machines, surgical instruments, and personal protective equipment (PPE).
4. Pharmaceutical Industry Support: Western democracies can offer support to Iran in developing and strengthening its pharmaceutical industry. This can involve sharing knowledge and best practices in pharmaceutical research and development, manufacturing processes, quality control, and regulatory compliance.
5. Access to Medicines: Western democracies can work with Iran to improve access to essential medicines. This can include capacity-building initiatives related to pharmaceutical supply chain management, distribution systems, and pricing mechanisms that ensure the affordability and availability of medicines for the Iranian population.
6. Research and Development Collaboration: Western democracies can collaborate with Iranian institutions and researchers on joint research projects and initiatives. This can include sharing expertise in medical research, clinical trials, drug discovery, and the development of innovative healthcare solutions.
7. Healthcare Policy and Governance: Western democracies can provide guidance and technical assistance in healthcare policy development and governance. This can

involve supporting the establishment of regulatory frameworks, health insurance systems, and healthcare financing mechanisms that promote equitable access to quality healthcare services.

8. Public Health Initiatives: Western democracies can assist in the implementation of public health initiatives in Iran. This can include supporting vaccination programs, disease surveillance systems, health promotion campaigns, and capacity-building in areas such as epidemiology and public health management.

9. Collaboration with International Organizations: Western democracies can facilitate collaboration between Iran and international organizations such as the World Health Organization (WHO) and the United Nations (UN). This can help Iran access global expertise, funding, and resources to address healthcare challenges and improve healthcare outcomes.

By providing support in these areas, western democracies can contribute to the development of a robust healthcare and pharmaceutical sector in Iran, improving healthcare access, quality, and outcomes for the Iranian population.

Appendix 1

1. Technical Assistance and Capacity Building: Western democracies can provide technical assistance and capacity-building programs to enhance the skills and knowledge of healthcare professionals in Iran. This can involve training programs, workshops, and knowledge-sharing initiatives in areas such as clinical practices, healthcare management, and public health.

2. Infrastructure Development: Western democracies can assist in the development and modernization of healthcare infrastructure in Iran. This can include supporting the construction and renovation of hospitals, clinics, and healthcare facilities, as well as providing expertise in healthcare facility design, equipment procurement, and management.

3. Medical Equipment and Supplies: Western democracies can contribute to the provision of essential medical equipment, supplies, and technologies. This can involve donating or subsidizing the purchase of medical equipment such as diagnostic tools, imaging machines, surgical instruments, and laboratory equipment.

4. Pharmaceutical Industry Support: Western democracies can offer support to Iran in developing and strengthening its pharmaceutical industry. This can include sharing expertise in pharmaceutical research and development, manufacturing processes, quality control, and regulatory compliance. Collaboration in areas such as drug discovery, clinical trials, and pharmaceutical production can also be facilitated.

5. Access to Medicines: Western democracies can work with Iran to improve access to affordable and quality medicines. This can involve supporting initiatives to

enhance pharmaceutical supply chains, improve distribution systems, and promote fair pricing mechanisms. Collaboration in areas such as generic medicine production and bulk procurement can also be explored.

6. Research and Development Collaboration: Western democracies can collaborate with Iranian institutions and researchers on joint research projects and initiatives. This can include sharing expertise in medical research, clinical trials, and the development of innovative healthcare solutions. Collaboration can also extend to areas such as epidemiology, public health research, and health technology innovation.

7. Policy and Regulatory Support: Western democracies can provide guidance and assistance in the development of healthcare policies, regulations, and standards. This can include support in areas such as healthcare financing, health insurance systems, regulatory frameworks, and quality assurance mechanisms. Collaboration can also extend to areas such as health information systems and data management.

8. Public Health Initiatives: Western democracies can support public health initiatives in Iran, such as disease prevention and control programs, vaccination campaigns, and health promotion initiatives. Collaboration can also involve sharing expertise in areas such as epidemiology, public health surveillance, and emergency preparedness.

9. Collaboration with International Organizations: Western democracies can facilitate collaboration between Iran and international organizations such as the World Health Organization (WHO) and the United Nations (UN). This can help Iran access global expertise, funding, and resources to address healthcare challenges and improve healthcare outcomes.

By providing support in these areas, western democracies can contribute to the development of a robust and sustainable healthcare and pharmaceutical sector in Iran, improving healthcare access, quality, and outcomes for the Iranian population.

Appendix 2

1. Training Programs: Western democracies can develop and deliver specialized training programs for healthcare professionals in Iran. These programs can focus on specific areas such as clinical skills, patient care, disease management, and healthcare technology. They can be designed to improve the practical skills and knowledge of healthcare professionals, equipping them with the latest advancements and best practices in their respective fields.

2. Workshops and Conferences: Western democracies can organize workshops and conferences in collaboration with Iranian healthcare institutions and professional associations. These events can provide opportunities for healthcare professionals to learn from experts, exchange ideas, and discuss emerging trends and challenges in their fields. They can also facilitate networking and collaboration among healthcare professionals from Iran and Western democracies.

3. Exchange Programs: Western democracies can establish exchange programs that allow healthcare professionals from Iran to visit and learn from healthcare institutions in Western democracies. These programs can provide firsthand exposure to advanced healthcare practices, innovative technologies, and research methodologies. They can also foster cross-cultural understanding and collaboration between healthcare professionals from different countries.

4. Mentoring and Coaching: Western democracies can facilitate mentorship and coaching programs for healthcare professionals in Iran. Experienced professionals from Western democracies can serve as mentors to guide and support their Iranian counterparts. This can involve regular meetings, discussions, and feedback sessions to help healthcare professionals enhance their skills, build confidence, and excel in their careers.

5. Online Learning Resources: Western democracies can develop and provide online learning resources, such as webinars, e-learning modules, and online courses, that are accessible to healthcare professionals in Iran. These resources can cover a wide range of topics, from clinical skills to healthcare management, allowing healthcare professionals to access learning materials at their own pace and convenience.

6. Research Collaboration: Western democracies can collaborate with Iranian healthcare institutions and researchers on joint research projects. This can involve sharing expertise, resources, and funding to conduct research studies that address healthcare challenges and contribute to scientific knowledge. Collaboration in research can enhance the research capabilities of healthcare professionals in Iran and foster innovation in healthcare practices.

7. Continuous Professional Development: Western democracies can support the establishment of continuous professional development programs for healthcare professionals in Iran. These programs can include ongoing training, workshops, and certifications that allow healthcare professionals to stay updated with the latest developments in their fields. Continuous professional development programs can help healthcare professionals maintain high standards of practice and provide quality care to patients.

By providing these types of assistance, Western democracies can contribute to the continuous professional growth and development of healthcare professionals in Iran, ultimately improving the quality of healthcare services and patient outcomes.

Appendix 3

1. Matching Mentors and Mentees: The program organizers can carefully match experienced mentors from Western democracies with healthcare professionals in Iran based on their areas of expertise, interests, and career goals. This ensures that mentees receive guidance and support from mentors who have relevant knowledge and experience.

2. Regular Meetings and Communication: Mentors and mentees can have regular meetings, either in person or through virtual platforms, to discuss career goals, challenges, and development opportunities. These meetings can be scheduled at regular intervals to provide ongoing support and guidance. Communication channels such as email, phone calls, or messaging apps can also be utilized for regular communication between mentors and mentees.
3. Goal Setting and Action Planning: Mentors can help mentees identify their career goals and create action plans to achieve them. They can assist mentees in setting specific, measurable, achievable, relevant, and time-bound (SMART) goals and guide the steps needed to reach those goals. Mentors can also help mentees navigate challenges and make informed decisions about their career paths.
4. Sharing Knowledge and Experience: Mentors can share their knowledge, expertise, and experiences with mentees, providing insights and guidance on various aspects of their profession. They can offer advice on clinical practices, research methodologies, leadership skills, and career advancement strategies. Mentors can also share relevant resources, such as articles, books, or online courses, to support the mentees' learning and development.
5. Providing Feedback and Support: Mentors can provide constructive feedback to mentees on their performance, skills, and areas for improvement. They can offer guidance and support in developing specific competencies and addressing any professional challenges mentees may face. Mentors can also serve as a sounding board for mentees, providing a safe space to discuss concerns, dilemmas, and career-related decisions.
6. Networking Opportunities: Mentors can help mentees expand their professional networks by introducing them to relevant contacts and connecting them with professional associations, conferences, and other networking events. Mentors can also provide recommendations or referrals to help mentees access career opportunities, collaborations, or further education.
7. Monitoring and Evaluation: Mentoring and coaching programs can include a monitoring and evaluation component to assess the effectiveness and impact of the program. Program organizers can collect feedback from both mentors and mentees to identify areas of improvement and make necessary adjustments to enhance the program's outcomes.
8. Ongoing Support and Alumni Engagement: Even after the formal mentoring period ends, mentors can continue to provide occasional support and guidance to mentees. Program organizers can also create alumni networks or platforms where mentees can connect and continue to share experiences, resources, and opportunities.

By implementing these strategies, mentoring and coaching programs can effectively support healthcare professionals in Iran, fostering their professional growth, and contributing to their success in the healthcare field.

Rebuilding Iran Healthcare Systems

Re-Engaging Female Healthcare Professionals: Addressing Gender Discrimination and Abuse in a Religious System

This report aims to provide a comprehensive analysis of the strategies and recommendations for re-engaging female healthcare professionals who have experienced gender discrimination and abuse in a religious system. The report seeks to address the challenges faced by these professionals and offer solutions to create an inclusive and supportive environment that promotes gender equality and empowers female healthcare professionals. By highlighting the root causes, identifying contributing factors, and proposing strategies, the report aims to facilitate positive change and ensure the re-engagement of female healthcare professionals in a religious system.

Introduction

Gender discrimination and abuse are pervasive issues that persist in various industries, including healthcare. Within a religious system, these challenges can be particularly complex and sensitive. This report aims to provide a comprehensive analysis of the strategies and recommendations for re-engaging female healthcare professionals who have experienced gender discrimination and abuse in a religious system. By addressing these issues, we can create an inclusive and supportive environment that promotes gender equality and empowers female healthcare professionals.

Understanding Gender Discrimination and Abuse in a Religious System:

Definition and Types of Discrimination: Define gender discrimination and its various forms, including unequal pay, limited career advancement opportunities, biased hiring practices, and disparities in resources and support.

Impact on Female Healthcare Professionals: Highlight the consequences of gender discrimination and abuse on the physical and mental well-being of female healthcare professionals. Discuss the potential negative effects on job satisfaction, productivity, and overall workforce diversity.

Identifying Root Causes and Contributing Factors:

Religious Beliefs and Traditions: Examine how religious beliefs and traditions can sometimes perpetuate gender inequalities and discriminatory practices within healthcare systems.

Patriarchal Structures and Power Dynamics: Analyze the impact of patriarchal structures and power dynamics within religious systems, which may contribute to the marginalization of female healthcare professionals.

Sociocultural Norms and Stereotypes: Discuss how sociocultural norms and stereotypes influence the perception and treatment of women in healthcare settings within religious systems.

Strategies for Re-Engaging Female Healthcare Professionals

Education and Awareness: Implement educational programs to raise awareness about gender discrimination, its impact on healthcare systems, and the importance of gender equality.

Policy and Legal Reforms: Advocate for policy and legal reforms that protect the rights of female healthcare professionals, including anti-discrimination laws, equal pay legislation, and workplace harassment policies.

Support Networks and Mentorship Programs: Establish support networks and mentorship programs to provide guidance, encouragement, and professional development opportunities for female healthcare professionals.

Cultural Sensitivity Training: Offer cultural sensitivity training to healthcare professionals and religious leaders to foster understanding, empathy, and respect for diverse perspectives and experiences.

Reporting Mechanisms and Support Services: Establish confidential reporting mechanisms and support services to encourage female healthcare professionals to come forward with their experiences of discrimination and abuse.

Addressing gender discrimination and abuse in a religious system requires a multi-faceted approach that involves education, policy reforms, support networks, and cultural sensitivity training. By implementing these strategies, healthcare systems can create an environment that promotes gender equality, supports the re-engagement of female healthcare professionals, and ensures the provision of high-quality care to all individuals, regardless of gender. It is crucial to continuously strive for inclusivity and equality in healthcare settings to create a fair and thriving workforce.

Female healthcare professionals within the religious system face several specific challenges, including:

1. Gender discrimination: They may experience discrimination based on their gender, which can manifest in various ways, such as unequal pay, limited career advancement opportunities, and a lack of recognition for their skills and contributions.

2. Limited leadership roles: Female healthcare professionals may face barriers in assuming leadership positions within the religious system. This can result in a lack ofrepresentation and decision-making power, hindering their ability to shape policies and practices that affect their work environment.

3. Cultural and religious expectations: The religious system may impose strict cultural and religious expectations on female healthcare professionals, which can conflict with their

professional aspirations and personal choices. This can include dress codes, restrictions on interactions with male colleagues or patients, and limitations on career choices.

4. Lack of support and mentorship: Female healthcare professionals may struggle to find adequate support and mentorship within the religious system. The absence of role models and mentors can hinder their professional development and growth, making it harder to navigate the challenges they face.

5. Harassment and abuse: Female healthcare professionals may be subjected to various forms of harassment and abuse, ranging from verbal harassment to sexual harassment. This can create a hostile work environment and negatively impact their physical and mental well-being.

It is important to note that these challenges can vary depending on the specific religious system and cultural context.

Some specific challenges faced by female healthcare professionals within the religious system include:

1. Limited access to education and training: Female healthcare professionals may face barriers in accessing quality education and training opportunities due to cultural and religious norms that prioritize male education. This can limit their ability to acquire the necessary skills and knowledge for their profession.

2. Gender bias and discrimination: Female healthcare professionals may experience gender bias and discrimination in the workplace, such as unequal pay, limited career advancement opportunities, and a lack of recognition for their expertise. This can hinder their professional growth and impact their overall job satisfaction.

3. Cultural and religious expectations: Female healthcare professionals within the religious system may be expected to adhere to strict cultural and religious norms, which can restrict their autonomy and decision-making abilities. This can include dress codes, restrictions on working with male colleagues or patients, and limitations on the types of procedures they can perform.

4. Balancing work and family responsibilities: Female healthcare professionals often face the challenge of balancing their professional responsibilities with their family and caregiving duties. This can be particularly challenging within the religious system, where traditional gender roles may place a greater emphasis on women's domestic responsibilities.

5. Lack of support and mentorship: Female healthcare professionals may struggle to find support and mentorship within the religious system, as they may have limited access to female role models and mentors who can guide and support their career development.

6. Ethical dilemmas: Female healthcare professionals within the religious system may encounter ethical dilemmas that are specific to their religious beliefs and practices. They

may be required to navigate situations where their professional obligations conflict with religious teachings or expectations.

It is important to recognize that these challenges can vary depending on the specific religious system and cultural context in which female healthcare professionals operate.

Female healthcare professionals may face several barriers in accessing education and training, including:

1. Cultural and societal norms: Some cultures and societies prioritize male education over female education, leading to limited opportunities for women to pursue higher education and professional training in healthcare fields. Gender biases and stereotypes can reinforce the perception that women are better suited for domestic roles rather than pursuing careers in healthcare.

2. Lack of resources: Limited financial resources can be a significant barrier for women seeking education and training in healthcare. Financial constraints may make it difficult for them to afford tuition fees, books, and other educational materials. This can prevent women from pursuing their desired healthcare professions or accessing higher-quality educational institutions.

3. Distance and transportation: In some regions, women may face challenges in accessing educational institutions due to geographical distances and limited transportation options. This can be particularly problematic for those living in rural areas or areas with inadequate infrastructure. The lack of safe and reliable transportation options may make it difficult for women to commute to educational institutions regularly.

4. Family and societal expectations: Societal and family expectations often place a greater emphasis on women's domestic roles and responsibilities, which can discourage them from pursuing higher education and professional training. Traditional gender roles and cultural norms may prioritize marriage and family over career aspirations, leading to societal pressure on women to prioritize these roles instead of pursuing their professional goals.

5. Gender discrimination and bias: Women may face discrimination and bias in educational institutions, including biased admission processes or limited opportunities for scholarships and grants. Stereotypes and biases may create a hostile learning environment that discourages women from pursuing education and training in healthcare fields.

6. Lack of female role models and mentors: The underrepresentation of women in leadership positions and faculty roles in healthcare education and training institutes can make it challenging for female healthcare professionals to find role models and mentors who can guide and support their educational journey. This lack of representation can hinder their motivation and confidence in pursuing their chosen healthcare professions.

Addressing these barriers requires comprehensive efforts, including promoting gender equality in education, providing financial support and scholarships for women in healthcare, improving transportation infrastructure, challenging gender stereotypes, and encouraging the presence of female role models and mentors in the field.

Some other specific challenges and barriers:

Family and societal expectations can have a significant impact on women's access to education and training in healthcare. These expectations often prioritize traditional gender roles and responsibilities, which can create barriers for women in pursuing their educational and professional aspirations in the healthcare field.

1. Limited support for education: In some cultures, and societies, there is a greater emphasis on women's domestic roles and responsibilities, such as marriage and raising a family. This can lead to limited support and encouragement for women to pursue higher education and professional training in healthcare. Families may prioritize early marriage or caregiving duties over investing in a woman's education, which can hinder her ability to access educational opportunities.

2. Pressure to conform to gender norms: Traditional gender norms and expectations may reinforce the idea that women should prioritize family and domestic responsibilities over career aspirations. This pressure to conform to societal expectations can discourage women from pursuing education and training in healthcare. They may face resistance or disapproval from family members or face societal judgments for deviating from the expected gender roles.

3. Lack of autonomy and decision-making power: In some societies, women may have limited autonomy and decision-making power when it comes to their education and career choices. Family members, particularly male relatives, may have the final say in determining a woman's educational path. This can result in women being discouraged or restricted from pursuing healthcare education and training, limiting their opportunities for professional growth.

4. Economic considerations: Family and societal expectations may prioritize economic considerations over women's education and career aspirations. Women may be expected to contribute to the family income or support the household through domestic work. This can lead to limited resources being allocated towards their education and training, making it difficult for them to access quality healthcare education.

5. Lack of role models and support networks: Family and societal expectations can also influence the availability of role models and support networks for women in healthcare. The underrepresentation of women in leadership positions and healthcare professions may limit the visibility of successful female healthcare professionals. Without visible role models and support networks, women may face challenges in navigating their educational and professional journeys.

Addressing these challenges requires challenging gender norms, promoting gender equality, and creating supportive environments that encourage women to pursue education and healthcare training. This can involve raising awareness about the importance of women's education, providing mentorship and support networks, and advocating for policies that promote women's access to education and career opportunities.

Furthermore, many of these combined factors are influenced by family, societal, cultural, and gender-specific economic dynamics. Here are some common and combined factors:

1. Gender expectations and traditional roles: Traditional gender roles and expectations often prioritize women's domestic responsibilities and caregiving roles. This can lead to limited support and encouragement for women to pursue higher education and professional training in healthcare. Family members or society may believe that a woman's primary role is to get married, raise a family, or provide domestic support, rather than focusing on a healthcare career.

2. Societal norms and stereotypes: Societal norms and stereotypes can create barriers for women in accessing education and training in healthcare. There may be a prevailing belief that certain professions, including healthcare, are more suitable for men, while women are expected to pursue careers in fields such as teaching or nursing. These stereotypes can discourage women from pursuing their interests and aspirations in healthcare.

3. Economic constraints: Economic constraints can limit women's access to higher education and professional training in healthcare. Financial resources may be limited within families, making it challenging to invest in a woman's education. In some cases, families prioritize investing in the education of male children over female children, perpetuating gender inequality in educational opportunities.

4. Lack of role models and support networks: The absence of visible role models and support networks in the healthcare field can discourage women from pursuing educational and professional pathways in healthcare. When women do not see other successful women in healthcare roles, they may feel discouraged or uncertain about their abilities to excel in this field. The lack of support networks can also make it difficult for women to navigate the challenges and barriers they may face.

5. Cultural and societal expectations: Cultural and societal expectations can play a significant role in limiting women's support and encouragement to pursue healthcare education and training. Cultural norms or religious beliefs may prioritize early marriage, motherhood, or familial duties over women's educational pursuits. These expectations can restrict women's autonomy and decision-making power regarding their career choices.

Addressing these factors requires concerted efforts to challenge gender stereotypes, promote gender equality, and create supportive environments. It involves raising awareness about the importance of women's education and career opportunities, providing mentorship and support networks, and advocating for policies that promote equal access to education and training in healthcare for women.

The absence of visible role models and support networks in the healthcare field can discourage women from pursuing educational and professional pathways in healthcare for several reasons:

1. Lack of representation: When women do not see other women in leadership positions or successful roles within the healthcare field, it can create a sense of invisibility and make it difficult for them to envision themselves in similar roles. Lack of representation can make it challenging for women to believe that they can succeed and excel in healthcare careers.

2. Limited mentorship opportunities: Role models often play a crucial role in providing guidance and mentorship to aspiring professionals. They can share their experiences, offer advice, and provide support throughout their educational and professional journey. Without visible role models, women may lack access to mentorship opportunities, which can hinder their personal and professional development.

3. Confidence and self-doubt: The absence of visible role models can contribute to feelings of self-doubt and low confidence among women considering a healthcare career. They may question their abilities and qualifications, wondering if they can succeed in a field where they do not see people like themselves thriving.

4. Perception of limited opportunities: Without visible role models, women may perceive limited opportunities for advancement and career growth in the healthcare field. This perception can discourage them from pursuing higher education and training, as they may believe that their efforts will not be recognized or rewarded.

5. Difficulty navigating challenges: Support networks are essential for navigating the challenges and barriers that may arise in any career path, including healthcare. Without access to support networks, women may find it more challenging to overcome obstacles, seek guidance, and find resources that can help them succeed.

To address these challenges, it is important to promote the visibility of women role models in the healthcare field. This can be achieved by highlighting the accomplishments and contributions of women in healthcare through media representation, professional networks, and mentorship programs. Creating support networks and mentorship opportunities specifically designed for women in healthcare can also provide the necessary guidance and encouragement for women to pursue educational and professional pathways in the field.

Solutions, Remedies, and Lessons Learned:

Separating religious doctrine from healthcare and medical education requires a commitment to providing evidence-based, patient-centered care while respecting individual beliefs and values. Here are some steps that can help in achieving this separation:

1. Emphasize scientific knowledge: Healthcare and medical education should prioritize scientific evidence, research, and best practices. Emphasize the importance of evidence-based medicine and critical thinking skills in decision-making processes. This ensures that medical professionals are equipped with the most accurate and up-to-date information.

2. Understand and respect diverse beliefs: Recognize that patients and healthcare professionals come from diverse religious and cultural backgrounds. Encourage an environment of respect and understanding for different beliefs and values.

3. Provide comprehensive education: Ensure that medical education includes comprehensive training on a wide range of medical topics, including reproductive health, end-of-life care, LGBTQ+ healthcare, and other areas that may intersect with religious beliefs. This education should be based on medical evidence and guidelines, rather than religious doctrine.

4. Encourage open dialogue: Create spaces for open and respectful dialogue among healthcare professionals, where they can discuss ethical dilemmas and navigate conflicts that may arise due to differing beliefs. This helps foster a healthcare environment that values diversity and promotes patient-centered care.

5. Maintain professional boundaries: Healthcare professionals should adhere to professional codes of ethics and maintain appropriate boundaries between their personal beliefs and the care they provide. While personal beliefs are important, they should not interfere with the provision of evidence-based, patient-centered care.

6. Establish clear policies: Healthcare institutions can develop clear policies that outline the separation of religious doctrine from healthcare practices. These policies should prioritize patient autonomy, informed consent, and the provision of unbiased care.

7. Provide resources for patients: Ensure that patients have access to unbiased information and resources that enable them to make informed decisions about their healthcare. This includes providing information about available healthcare options, potential risks and benefits, and alternative treatments.

By prioritizing evidence-based medicine, respecting diverse beliefs, and promoting open dialogue, healthcare and medical education can effectively separate religious doctrine from the provision of healthcare services. This approach ensures that patients receive the best possible care while respecting their values and beliefs.

Procedures and Materials:

Achieving the separation of religious doctrine from healthcare and medical education requires a multifaceted approach. Here are some steps that can help in achieving this goal:

1. Establish clear guidelines and policies: Healthcare institutions and educational organizations should develop clear guidelines and policies that outline the separation of religious doctrine from healthcare and medical education. These policies should prioritize evidence-based practices, patient autonomy, and the provision of unbiased care.

2. Emphasize evidence-based medicine: Healthcare and medical education should prioritize scientific evidence, research, and best practices. Emphasize the importance of

basing medical decisions on reliable evidence and critical thinking skills. This ensures that medical professionals are equipped with the most accurate and up-to-date information.

3. Provide comprehensive education: Ensure that medical education includes comprehensive training on a wide range of medical topics, including those that may intersect with religious beliefs. This includes reproductive health, end-of-life care, LGBTQ+ healthcare, and other sensitive areas. Education should be based on medical evidence and guidelines, rather than religious doctrine.

4. Foster an inclusive and respectful environment: Create an environment that values diversity and respects the beliefs and values of both healthcare professionals and patients. Encourage open dialogue and understanding of different perspectives. This can be achieved through workshops, cultural competency training, and promoting respectful communication.

5. Encourage critical thinking and ethical decision-making: Medical education should emphasize critical thinking skills and ethical decision-making processes. This helps healthcare professionals navigate complex situations where religious beliefs may intersect with medical care. Encourage professionals to consider the best interests of the patient while respecting their beliefs.

6. Support patient autonomy and informed consent: Prioritize patient autonomy by ensuring that patients have access to unbiased information and resources. This includes providing information about available healthcare options, potential risks and benefits, and alternative treatments. Encourage healthcare professionals to engage in shared decision-making with their patients, respecting their values and preferences.

7. Maintain professional boundaries: Healthcare professionals should adhere to professional codes of ethics and maintain appropriate boundaries between their personal beliefs and the care they provide. While personal beliefs are important, they should not interfere with the provision of evidence-based, patient-centered care.

By implementing these steps, healthcare and medical education can effectively separate religious doctrine from the provision of healthcare services. This approach ensures that patients receive the best possible care while respecting their values and beliefs.

It is important for healthcare and medical education to prioritize evidence-based practices and patient autonomy for several reasons:

1. Ensuring the best outcomes: Evidence-based practices are rooted in scientific research and are effective in improving patient outcomes. By prioritizing evidence-based practices, healthcare professionals can provide the most effective and efficient care to their patients. This leads to better health outcomes and improved quality of life.

2. Minimizing harm: Evidence-based practices are designed to minimize harm and reduce unnecessary risks to patients. They are based on rigorous research, clinical trials, and

systematic reviews of the available evidence. By following evidence-based guidelines, healthcare professionals can minimize the potential for medical errors, adverse events, and unnecessary procedures.

3. Promoting efficiency and cost-effectiveness: Evidence-based practices help healthcare institutions make informed decisions about resource allocation and utilization. By focusing on interventions with proven effectiveness, healthcare providers can optimize the use of limited resources and reduce unnecessary healthcare costs. This is especially important in today's healthcare landscape, where resources are often constrained.

4. Respecting patient autonomy: Patient autonomy is the right of patients to make informed decisions about their healthcare, based on their values, preferences, and goals. By prioritizing patient autonomy, healthcare professionals empower patients to actively participate in their care. This involves providing them with accurate and unbiased information, involving them in shared decision-making, and respecting their choices.

5. Upholding ethical principles: Prioritizing evidence-based practices and patient autonomy aligns with fundamental ethical principles in healthcare, such as beneficence, non-maleficence, and respect for autonomy. It ensures that healthcare professionals act in the best interest of their patients, respect their values and preferences, and avoid imposing their own beliefs or biases onto patients.

6. Fostering trust and transparency: By prioritizing evidence-based practices and patient autonomy, healthcare institutions and professionals demonstrate their commitment to providing high-quality, patient-centered care. This fosters trust between patients and healthcare providers, as patients can have confidence that their care is based on the best available evidence and that their values and preferences are respected.

Overall, prioritizing evidence-based practices and patient autonomy in healthcare and medical education is essential for improving patient outcomes, minimizing harm, promoting efficiency, respecting ethical principles, and fostering trust. It ensures that healthcare decisions are grounded in scientific evidence and that patients are active participants in their care.

Changing Healthcare and New Paradigm:

The fundamental ethical principle in healthcare that recognizes a person's right to make decisions about their healthcare is "respect for autonomy." This principle acknowledges that individuals have the right to make decisions about their own bodies, health, and medical treatment. It involves respecting and supporting patients' ability to make informed choices based on their values, beliefs, and preferences. Healthcare professionals uphold this principle by providing patients with accurate information, involving them in shared decision-making, and respecting their decisions, even if they differ from the healthcare professional's recommendations. Respect for autonomy is a cornerstone of patient-centered care and is essential for promoting individual rights and dignity in healthcare.

Prioritizing patient autonomy in healthcare aligns with several ethical principles, including:

1. Respect for autonomy: Respect for autonomy is a fundamental ethical principle in healthcare that recognizes a person's right to make decisions about their healthcare. By prioritizing patient autonomy, healthcare professionals acknowledge and respect the individual's right to make choices based on their values, beliefs, and preferences. This includes providing patients with accurate information, involving them in shared decision-making, and respecting their decisions, even if they differ from the healthcare professional's recommendations.

2. Beneficence: Beneficence is the ethical principle that emphasizes the duty to act in the best interest of the patient. Prioritizing patient autonomy aligns with beneficence by recognizing that patients are in the best position to determine what is in their own best interest. By respecting and supporting their autonomy, healthcare professionals can ensure that interventions and treatment plans are aligned with the patient's preferences and goals, ultimately promoting their well-being.

3. Non-maleficence: Non-maleficence is the principle that emphasizes the obligation to not harm the patient. Prioritizing patient autonomy helps prevent harm by ensuring that healthcare decisions and interventions are made with the patient's informed consent. By involving patients in the decision-making process, healthcare professionals can better understand their values, preferences, and potential concerns, allowing them to minimize the risk of harm and avoid imposing unwanted or unnecessary interventions.

4. Justice: Justice is the principle that focuses on fairness and equitable distribution of healthcare resources. Prioritizing patient autonomy helps uphold justice by treating each patient as an individual with unique needs, values, and preferences. It ensures that healthcare decisions are not based on arbitrary criteria or biased judgments but rather on the specific circumstances and wishes of the patient. This promotes fairness and equality in the provision of healthcare services.

5. Transparency and trust: Prioritizing patient autonomy promotes transparency and trust in the patient-provider relationship. By involving patients in the decision-making process, healthcare professionals demonstrate respect, openness, and honesty. This fosters trust between the patient and healthcare provider, as patients feel empowered and supported in making decisions about their care. Transparent communication and shared decision-making build a strong foundation for a trusting and collaborative relationship.

In summary, prioritizing patient autonomy in healthcare aligns with ethical principles such as respect for autonomy, beneficence, non-maleficence, justice, and transparency. It recognizes and respects the patient's rights, promotes their well-being, minimizes harm, ensures fairness, and fosters trust in the patient-provider relationship. By upholding these ethical principles, healthcare professionals can provide patient-centered care that respects the autonomy and values of everyone.

Religions, Progress Perspectives, and Reality State of Mind, Beliefs or Brainwash

Stagnant Strongholds: Identifying Religions Hindering Progress

Religious doctrine, like any belief system, can have a wide range of effects on individuals' thinking and intellectual development. It is important to note that not all religious doctrines promote simplemindedness or discourage higher thinking.

Religious doctrines often include moral and ethical teachings, guide how to live a meaningful life, and offer explanations about the nature of the world and existence. They can serve as sources of inspiration, comfort, and community for many people.

However, some interpretations or practices of religious doctrines may discourage critical thinking or discourage questioning of established beliefs. This can potentially limit intellectual exploration and inhibit the development of independent thought. In such cases, individuals may rely solely on religious teachings without critically examining or engaging with alternative perspectives or knowledge from other fields.

It is worth mentioning that many religious traditions have a rich history of intellectual thought, scholarly inquiry, and philosophical discourse. Throughout history, religious institutions and thinkers have made significant contributions to various fields such as science, philosophy, and the arts. Many religious individuals also engage in deep intellectual exploration while maintaining their faith.

Ultimately, the impact of religious doctrine on thinking and intellectual development varies widely depending on factors such as individual interpretation, cultural context, and the openness of the religious community to intellectual inquiry. It is important to approach discussions on this topic with nuance, recognizing the diversity of beliefs and experiences within religious communities.

The belief in an afterlife and the concept of living in heaven can have both positive and negative impacts on society and cultural development. While it is important to acknowledge that these impacts can vary depending on individual beliefs and interpretations, here are some potential negative effects:

1. Devaluation of the Present: The belief in a heavenly afterlife can sometimes lead to a devaluation of the present life and a focus on the rewards and pleasures of the afterlife. This may result in a diminished emphasis on improving the current society and culture, as some individuals may prioritize their spiritual journey and eternal salvation over worldly matters.
2. Fatalism and Inaction: The belief in a heavenly afterlife can sometimes lead to a sense of fatalism, where individuals may believe that the ultimate salvation lies in

the afterlife and that worldly problems are inconsequential. This can discourage active engagement in social, cultural, and political issues, potentially hindering progress and development.

3. Intolerance and Exclusivity: The belief in a specific afterlife, exclusive to a particular religious group, can foster a sense of religious exclusivity and intolerance towards those who hold different beliefs. This can lead to social divisions, conflicts, and a lack of cultural diversity and inclusivity.
4. Suppression of Critical Thinking: Some religious beliefs about the afterlife may discourage questioning or challenging the established doctrines and authorities. This can hinder intellectual curiosity, scientific progress, and cultural innovation, as individuals may be discouraged from exploring new ideas that challenge traditional religious teachings.
5. Neglect of Earthly Responsibilities: The preoccupation with the afterlife and heavenly rewards can sometimes lead to a neglect of earthly responsibilities, such as social justice, environmental stewardship, and the well-being of the present society. This can hinder social progress and cultural development as individuals may prioritize spiritual pursuits over addressing pressing societal issues.
6. It is important to note that these negative impacts do not apply to all individuals or religious beliefs. The interpretation and practice of the belief in an afterlife can vary greatly, and many religious traditions also emphasize the importance of social responsibility, justice, and compassion in the present life.

The concepts of heaven and hell, as presented in some religious doctrines, can have varying effects on individuals' thinking and attitudes towards life. It is important to note that different religious traditions have different interpretations of heaven and hell, and individuals within those traditions may hold diverse beliefs.

For some individuals, the belief in heaven and hell can provide a sense of purpose, hope, and moral guidance. It can serve as a motivation to live a virtuous life and strive for spiritual growth. The concept of an afterlife can also offer comfort in times of hardship or loss.

However, in certain cases, the belief in heaven and hell can potentially discourage critical thinking and lead to a devaluation of the present life. Some individuals may focus primarily on the rewards and punishments of the afterlife, which can diminish the importance of personal growth, ethical decision-making, and social responsibility in the present moment. This mindset may lead to a passive acceptance of the status quo or a disregard for addressing societal issues.

Moreover, the belief in an eternal afterlife can create a tendency to prioritize the future over the present, potentially leading to a neglect of personal and social well-being in the here and now. This may result in a reluctance to question existing power structures, challenge social norms, or actively seek improvement in the current world.

It is essential to recognize that not all individuals within religious communities interpret or apply the concept of heaven and hell in the same way. Many religious individuals find a balance between their belief in an afterlife and their engagement with critical thinking, personal growth, and making a positive impact in the present world.

Ultimately, the influence of the concept of heaven and hell on critical thinking and acceptance of minimalism in life can vary significantly among individuals and religious communities. It is important to approach this topic with respect for diverse beliefs and to encourage open dialogue that promotes both spiritual exploration and intellectual inquiry.

SIMPLICITY OF MIND

Simplicity of mind refers to a state of having a straightforward and uncomplicated approach to thinking and perceiving the world. It is often associated with innocence, naivety, and a lack of complexity in thought processes. On the other hand, abuse refers to the mistreatment, harm, or exploitation of someone, either physically, emotionally, or psychologically.

The relationship between simplicity of mind and abuse can be complex. While simplicity of mind can make an individual more vulnerable to abuse, it is important to note that abuse can happen to anyone regardless of their level of complexity in thinking. Here are a few key points to consider:

1. Vulnerability: Individuals with a simple or uncomplicated mindset may be more susceptible to manipulation and exploitation. Their trusting nature and lack of skepticism can make them an easy target for those seeking to take advantage of them. This vulnerability can manifest in various forms of abuse, including emotional manipulation, financial exploitation, or even physical harm.
2. Lack of awareness: Simplicity of mind may lead to a limited understanding of abusive behaviors or recognition of red flags. Individuals with a straightforward approach to thinking may struggle to recognize signs of abuse or may be more inclined to dismiss or overlook problematic behaviors. This lack of awareness can prolong the abuse and prevent the individual from seeking help or taking appropriate action.
3. Power dynamics: Abuse often involves an imbalance of power, with the abuser exerting control over the victim. Individuals with a simple mindset may be more submissive and less likely to challenge or question the authority of the abuser. This power imbalance can make it difficult for them to escape the abusive situation or seek support.
4. Societal norms and expectations: Simplicity of mind can be influenced by societal norms and expectations that promote obedience, compliance, and conformity. These norms may discourage individuals from questioning abusive behaviors or seeking

help, further perpetuating the cycle of abuse.

5. It is important to emphasize that the vulnerability associated with simplicity of mind does not justify or excuse abuse in any way. Abuse is never acceptable or justified regardless of an individual's mindset or level of complexity in thinking. It is crucial to raise awareness about abuse, promote education and empowerment, and provide support systems for individuals who may be vulnerable to or experiencing abuse, regardless of their mindset.

Simplicity of mind can impact an individual's ability to recognize signs of abuse or red flags in several ways:

1. Limited understanding: Individuals with a simple mindset may have a limited understanding of abusive behaviors and their consequences. They may lack knowledge about different forms of abuse, such as emotional manipulation, gaslighting, or coercive control. This limited understanding can make it difficult for them to recognize when they are being mistreated or manipulated.

2. Trusting nature: Simplicity of mind often involves a trusting and optimistic outlook on life. While this can be a positive trait, it can also make individuals more vulnerable to manipulation and exploitation. They may have difficulty suspecting or questioning the intentions of others, even when faced with concerning behaviors. This trusting nature can prevent them from recognizing red flags and taking necessary precautions.

3. Lack of skepticism: Individuals with simplicity of mind may tend to see the best in others and may be less inclined to be skeptical or suspicious. This lack of skepticism can make it challenging for them to question the motives or actions of someone who may be engaging in abusive behavior. They may give the benefit of the doubt even when faced with warning signs.

4. Difficulty in asserting boundaries: Those with simplicity of mind may struggle to assert their boundaries or recognize when their boundaries are being violated. They may be more accommodating and willing to overlook behaviors that infringe upon their personal space, emotional well-being, or autonomy. This difficulty in setting and enforcing boundaries can make it easier for abusers to continue their harmful actions unchecked.

5. 5. Overlooking problematic behaviors: Individuals with simplicity of mind may be inclined to overlook or dismiss problematic behaviors, attributing them to misunderstandings or giving others the benefit of the doubt. They may struggle to see patterns of abusive behavior or may rationalize and make excuses for the actions of the abuser. This can prevent them from recognizing the severity of the situation and seeking help.

6. Furthermore, It is important to note that while simplicity of mind can impact an individual's ability to recognize signs of abuse or red flags, it does not mean that

they are at fault or responsible for the abuse. Abusers are the ones who are accountable for their actions, and support and resources should be available to individuals who may be vulnerable to or experiencing abuse, regardless of their mindset.

The simplicity of mind and religious superstition can sometimes be interconnected, but it's important to approach this topic with sensitivity and respect for diverse beliefs and perspectives.

The simplicity of mind, which refers to a straightforward and uncomplicated way of thinking, can make individuals more susceptible to accepting and adhering to religious superstitions. This can occur when individuals have a limited understanding of scientific or rational explanations and rely more on beliefs, traditions, or supernatural explanations to make sense of the world. They may find comfort and security in following religious rituals, traditions, or superstitions without questioning their validity or seeking alternative explanations.

Religious superstitions are often based on cultural or religious beliefs that are not supported by empirical evidence or logical reasoning. They can include practices like avoiding certain actions or objects believed to bring bad luck, seeking divine intervention for everyday matters, or attributing events to supernatural causes. While some people may find solace or a sense of meaning in these beliefs, others may view them as irrational or unnecessary.

It's important to remember that beliefs and practices related to religion are deeply personal and can vary greatly across individuals and cultures. While simplicity of mind may make individuals more prone to accepting religious superstitions, it is not a universal characteristic of all religious individuals. Many religious individuals have complex and nuanced understandings of their faith and engage critically with their beliefs.

It is essential to approach discussions about religious beliefs and superstitions with empathy, respect, and an openness to understanding different perspectives. It is also important to recognize that individuals have the right to their own beliefs and should not be judged solely based on their level of simplicity of mind or adherence to superstitions.

ILLITERACY

Simplicity of mind and illiteracy are two different concepts that should not be equated or used interchangeably.

Simplicity of mind refers to a straightforward and uncomplicated way of thinking, often characterized by a lack of complexity or sophistication in one's thoughts and beliefs. It does not necessarily imply a lack of education or knowledge. Some individuals with a simplicity of mind may have a limited understanding of complex concepts or lack exposure to diverse perspectives, but this does not necessarily mean they are illiterate.

Illiteracy, on the other hand, refers to the inability to read or write. It is a lack of basic literacy skills and can significantly impact an individual's ability to access and understand written information. Illiteracy can be a result of limited educational opportunities, lack of access to quality education, or other socio-economic factors.

It's important to note that simplicity of mind and illiteracy are not mutually exclusive. While illiterate individuals may have limited exposure to formal education and complex ideas, it does not automatically mean they possess a simplicity of mind. Similarly, individuals with a simplicity of mind may or may not be literate.

It is crucial to address illiteracy by promoting accessible and quality education for all individuals. Education not only enhances literacy skills but also fosters critical thinking, creativity, and the ability to engage with diverse perspectives. However, it is essential to approach discussions about simplicity of mind and illiteracy with empathy and avoid making assumptions or generalizations about individuals based on their educational background or thought processes.

It's important to recognize that individuals can be both literate and have a simpleminded approach, or they can be illiterate but possess a more complex way of thinking. These are separate aspects of a person's cognitive abilities and should be considered independently.

Promoting literacy and providing quality education can help individuals enhance their reading and writing skills, while also fostering critical thinking and the ability to engage with more complex ideas. However, it is important to approach discussions about simplemindedness and illiteracy with sensitivity and avoid making assumptions or generalizations about individuals based solely on their educational background or thought processes.

DO SCIENCE AND RELIGIONS SEE EYE TO EYE?

GALILEO CONFLICT

Religions and Galileo's discoveries about the Earth have a complex historical relationship. In the 17th century, Galileo Galilei, an Italian astronomer and physicist, made significant observations and arguments supporting the heliocentric model of the solar system, which stated that the Earth revolves around the Sun. This challenged the prevailing geocentric model supported by the Catholic Church, which positioned Earth as the center of the universe.

Galileo's findings and his support for the heliocentric model brought him into conflict with the Church, which considered his ideas as contradicting the biblical interpretation of Earth's position and movement. Galileo faced opposition and was eventually put on trial by the Inquisition, leading to his recantation of his heliocentric views under threat of punishment.

It is important to note that the Church's reaction to Galileo's discoveries was not a reflection of all religious beliefs or all religious institutions. While the Catholic Church at the time held considerable influence, religious perspectives on scientific discoveries can vary among different faith traditions. Additionally, the Church's opposition to Galileo was not solely based on religious grounds but also involved complex political and institutional factors.

Over time, attitudes toward science and its relationship with religious beliefs have evolved. Many religious denominations and scholars have embraced scientific advancements, recognizing that scientific inquiry and religious faith can coexist and complement each other. Today, numerous religious groups accept the scientific consensus on the heliocentric model of the solar system and acknowledge the value of scientific exploration and understanding of the natural world.

Islam as a religion does not have a unified or official stance on scientific discoveries, including those made by Galileo Galilei. Islam emphasizes the pursuit of knowledge and encourages Muslims to explore and understand the natural world. Throughout history, there have been Muslim scholars who have embraced scientific advancements, while others may have held differing views.

It is worth noting that Galileo's discoveries and the heliocentric model of the solar system were met with opposition from various religious and scientific communities during his time, including within the Catholic Church. However, it is not accurate to make a blanket statement about Islam's position on Galileo's discoveries, as interpretations and attitudes can vary among individuals and communities within the religion

It is essential to recognize that religion and science address different aspects of human experience. While religion often deals with questions of meaning, purpose, and moral values, science focuses on empirical observations, experimentation, and the understanding of the natural world. Both can contribute to a comprehensive understanding of the universe, and many individuals integrate their religious beliefs with scientific knowledge in a harmonious way.

RELIGIOUS DISCRIMINATIONS:

Fighting against religious discrimination requires a collective effort from individuals, communities, organizations, and governments. Here are some steps that can be taken:

1. Education and Awareness: Promote education and awareness about different religions and beliefs to foster understanding, empathy, and tolerance. Encourage learning about diverse cultures and religions to challenge stereotypes and misconceptions.

2. Promote Dialogue and Interfaith Cooperation: Encourage open and respectful dialogue between individuals of different faiths. Foster interfaith cooperation and collaboration to promote understanding, bridge differences, and work towards common goals.

3. Advocate for Legal Protections: Support and advocate for laws and policies that protect individuals from religious discrimination. Work towards the implementation and enforcement of existing anti-discrimination laws.
4. Support Victims and Provide Resources: Offer support and resources to individuals who have experienced religious discrimination. Provide avenues for reporting incidents and ensure that victims have access to legal assistance, counseling, and other necessary support services.
5. Foster Inclusive Communities: Encourage the creation of inclusive communities that embrace diversity and respect different religious beliefs. Promote intercultural and interfaith events, celebrations, and initiatives that bring people together.
6. Challenge Stereotypes and Prejudice: Speak out against stereotypes, prejudice, and hate speech targeting individuals based on their religion. Promote media literacy and critical thinking to counter misinformation and promote understanding.
7. Engage in Peacebuilding and Conflict Resolution: Support initiatives that promote peacebuilding and conflict resolution, particularly in areas where religious tensions exist. Foster dialogue and mediation to address underlying issues and promote reconciliation.

ISLAM, ISLAMIC REPUBLIC AND WOMEN:

The vulnerability of women in civil struggles is a significant concern that deserves attention. When civil struggles or conflicts arise, women often face unique challenges and are disproportionately affected in various ways. Here are some key aspects of their vulnerability:

1. Gender-based violence: Women are at an increased risk of experiencing gender-based violence during civil struggles. This includes physical, sexual, and psychological violence perpetrated by both state and non-state actors. Sexual violence is often used as a weapon of war or a means to exert power and control over women. The trauma and long-term consequences of such violence can be devastating.
2. Displacement and instability: Women are more likely to be displaced from their homes and communities during civil struggles. This displacement can lead to loss of livelihoods, separation from family members, and increased vulnerability to exploitation and abuse. In refugee camps or temporary shelters, women may face inadequate access to healthcare, sanitation facilities, and protection from violence.
3. Limited access to resources and services: Women often face barriers in accessing basic resources and services during civil struggles. This can include limited access to food, water, healthcare, education, and economic opportunities. The disruption of infrastructure and institutions further exacerbates these challenges, making it harder for women to meet their basic needs and support themselves and their families.

4. Marginalization and exclusion: Women's voices and perspectives are often marginalized or excluded in decision-making processes during civil struggles. Their participation in peace negotiations, conflict resolution, and post-conflict reconstruction efforts is crucial for sustainable peace and inclusive societies. However, women are frequently underrepresented in these processes, limiting their ability to shape the outcomes and address their specific needs and concerns.
5. Disruption of social support systems: Civil struggles can disrupt traditional social support systems that women rely on, such as family networks, community structures, and support services. This can further isolate and marginalize women, leaving them without adequate support systems to address their physical, emotional, and economic needs.
6. Addressing the vulnerability of women in civil struggles requires a comprehensive approach that includes ensuring their safety and protection, promoting gender equality, supporting access to resources and services, and amplifying their voices and participation in decision-making processes. It is essential to recognize and address the unique challenges faced by women in civil struggles to create more inclusive and equitable societies.

Supporting women in civil struggles is crucial for several reasons:

1. Upholding human rights: Access to basic resources and services is a fundamental human right. By addressing the limited access faced by women in civil struggles, we ensure that their rights are upheld and protected. This includes access to food, water, healthcare, education, and economic opportunities. Denying women access to these essential resources not only violates their rights but also perpetuates inequality and reinforces their vulnerability.
2. Promoting gender equality: Limited access to resources and services often stems from gender inequalities and discriminatory practices. By addressing these barriers, we work towards achieving gender equality. When women have equal access to resources and services, they are better able to fulfill their potential, contribute to society, and participate in decision-making processes. Gender equality benefits not only women but also their families, communities, and society.
3. Enhancing resilience and recovery: Women play a crucial role in the recovery and rebuilding process after civil struggles. When women have access to resources and services, they can actively participate in rebuilding their lives and communities. This strengthens their resilience and contributes to the overall recovery and stability of the society. Women's participation in post-conflict reconstruction efforts is vital for creating sustainable peace and ensuring that the specific needs and priorities of women are addressed.
4. Breaking the cycle of poverty: Limited access to resources and services can perpetuate the cycle of poverty for women in civil struggles. When women are denied access to

education, economic opportunities, and social support, it becomes challenging for them to improve their socio-economic status. By addressing these barriers and providing equal opportunities, we can break the cycle of poverty and empower women to become economically independent and self-sufficient.

5. Building inclusive and equitable societies: Addressing the limited access to resources and services faced by women in civil struggles is essential for building inclusive and equitable societies. It ensures that no one is left behind and that women have equal opportunities to thrive and contribute to their communities. Inclusive societies are more resilient, peaceful, and just, benefiting everyone. By addressing the limited access to resources and services faced by women in their civil struggles, we not only uphold their rights and promote gender equality but also contribute to the overall well-being and development of societies. It is a necessary step towards creating a more just and inclusive world.

HOW TO INITIATE THE POLITICAL REFORM AND DEMOCRACY:

The principle of civil disobedience, also known as social disobedience, is a concept that promotes nonviolent resistance to challenge unjust laws, policies, or practices. It is rooted in the belief that individuals have a moral duty to act against injustice, even if it means disobeying certain laws or authorities.

The principles of social disobedience include:

1. Nonviolence: Civil disobedience is based on the principle of nonviolence. It emphasizes peaceful and nonviolent means to challenge injustice. This principle aims to maintain the moral high ground while advocating for change.

2. Conscientious Objection: Social disobedience is driven by a deep personal conviction and conscience. Individuals who engage in civil disobedience believe that certain laws or policies are morally wrong and feel compelled to take a stand against them.

3. Public Awareness and Education: Civil disobedience aims to raise public awareness about the issue at hand. By engaging in acts of disobedience, individuals seek to draw attention to the injustice, spark public dialogue, and educate others about the cause.

4. Acceptance of Legal Consequences: Those who practice civil disobedience are willing to accept the legal consequences of their actions. They understand that their actions may result in arrest, fines, or other penalties, but they believe that the greater cause justifies these consequences.

5. Respect for the Rule of Law: Civil disobedience does not seek to undermine the rule of law but rather to challenge unjust laws or practices within the existing legal framework. It acknowledges the importance of a just and fair legal system while

advocating for change.

6. Democratic Participation: Social disobedience is often rooted in democratic principles. It recognizes that individuals have the right to participate in shaping their society and that peaceful dissent is a legitimate form of political expression.
7. Collective Action: Civil disobedience often involves collective action and mobilization. It encourages individuals to come together, form alliances, and work collectively to challenge unjust laws or policies. This collective action enhances the impact and effectiveness of civil disobedience.

One of the key principles of civil disobedience that promotes public dialogue and education is the principle of public awareness and education. This principle emphasizes the importance of raising awareness about the issue at hand and educating the public about the cause for which civil disobedience is being practiced.

When engaging in civil disobedience, individuals intentionally draw attention to the injustice they are challenging. They aim to spark public dialogue and encourage discussions about the underlying issues. By bringing attention to the unjust laws, policies, or practices, civil disobedience seeks to create a platform for open and informed conversations.

Through acts of civil disobedience, individuals often use symbolic actions, protests, or demonstrations to capture public attention. These actions are designed to provoke thought, curiosity, and engagement among the public. They aim to create a space for dialogue and debate, where people can exchange ideas, share perspectives, and deepen their understanding of the issue.

Furthermore, civil disobedience often involves the dissemination of information, facts, and personal stories to educate the public about the cause. This can be done through various means such as public speeches, media interviews, social media campaigns, or the distribution of educational materials. By providing information and promoting understanding, civil disobedience seeks to empower individuals to form their own opinions and take informed action.

The principle of public awareness and education in civil disobedience recognizes that change cannot occur without the engagement and support of the wider public. By promoting dialogue and education, civil disobedience strives to build a broad-based movement for social change, encouraging individuals to question existing norms, challenge injustice, and contribute to a more informed and just society

It is important to note that civil disobedience should be undertaken responsibly and with careful consideration of the potential consequences. The principles of social disobedience promote peaceful resistance and aim to bring about positive social change while upholding the values of justice, equality, and human rights.

AND NEXT:

Mass Mobilization

The combination of mass mobilization tactics, such as protests, civil disobedience, and strikes, can lead to significant societal change and the shaping of destinies in several ways.

Firstly, mass mobilization creates a visible and powerful force that cannot be ignored by those in power. When large numbers of people come together to express their grievances and demand change, it sends a clear message that the current situation is no longer acceptable. This can put pressure on authorities to address the demands of the people and initiate reforms. Secondly, mass mobilization fosters a sense of unity and solidarity among the participants. When people join in protests or strikes, they realize that they are not alone in their struggles and that their voices matter. This collective consciousness can inspire individuals to take further action and engage in ongoing activism, leading to sustained efforts for change.

Additionally, mass mobilization can disrupt the normal functioning of society and the economy. Strikes, for example, can paralyze industries and force authorities to negotiate with workers and address their grievances. This disruption can create a sense of urgency and compel those in power to respond to restore stability.

Furthermore, mass mobilization can have a ripple effect on public opinion and discourse. When large-scale protests and acts of civil disobedience garner media attention and public support, they can shift the narrative and change societal perceptions. This can lead to a broader understanding of the issues at hand and generate momentum for change.

Lastly, the combination of mass mobilization tactics allows for diverse voices and perspectives to be heard. It brings people from different backgrounds and walks of life together, fostering a sense of inclusivity and representation. This diversity strengthens the movement and ensures that a wide range of concerns and demands are addressed, leading to more comprehensive and transformative societal change.

Overall, by combining mass mobilization tactics and mass education, societies could create significant change, challenge existing power structures, and shape their destinies.

چو ایران نباشد تن من مباد

بدین مرز و بوم زنده یک تن مباد

Remedy and Rebuilding: Restoring Hope and Professional Self-Worth

Introduction:

The healthcare system plays a crucial role in ensuring the well-being and quality of life of a nation's citizens. However, in the Islamic Republic of Iran, the healthcare system has been plagued by mismanagement, leading to a wide range of challenges. This essay will examine the key issues contributing to healthcare system mismanagement in Iran and suggest possible solutions to address these pressing concerns.

Inadequate Funding:

One of the primary causes of healthcare system mismanagement in Iran is the inadequate funding allocated to the sector. The government's budget for healthcare has consistently fallen short of meeting the growing demands and needs of the population. Insufficient funds lead to a scarcity of medical equipment, a shortage of qualified healthcare professionals, and inadequate infrastructure, all of which negatively impact the delivery of healthcare services to the Iranian people.

Brain Drain:

Another significant challenge faced by Iran's healthcare system is the phenomenon of brain drain. Skilled and highly qualified medical professionals are leaving the country in search of better opportunities abroad. This exodus of talent further exacerbates the shortage of healthcare professionals within the country. As a result, the remaining healthcare workforce is burdened with heavy workloads, leading to decreased efficiency and compromised patient care.

Lack of Accessible Healthcare:

Access to quality healthcare is a fundamental right of every citizen. However, in Iran, the lack of accessible healthcare services is a major concern. Rural areas suffer from inadequate healthcare infrastructure, limited medical facilities, and a scarcity of healthcare professionals. This imbalance in healthcare distribution leaves a significant portion of the population without proper access to timely and affordable healthcare services, leading to worsened health outcomes and disparities.

Corruption and Misallocation of Resources:

Corruption within the healthcare system further contributes to its mismanagement in Iran. Reports of embezzlement, bribery

Inadequate funding has a profound impact on the delivery of healthcare services in Iran. Here are some key ways in which inadequate funding affects the healthcare system:

1. Limited Medical Equipment and Supplies: Insufficient funds result in a scarcity of essential medical equipment and supplies. Hospitals and healthcare facilities struggle to acquire and maintain the necessary equipment, such as diagnostic tools, surgical instruments, and life-saving machinery. This shortage hampers the ability of healthcare providers to deliver timely and effective treatments, leading to compromised patient care.

2. Shortage of Healthcare Professionals: Inadequate funding also contributes to a shortage of qualified healthcare professionals. Healthcare providers are unable to offer competitive salaries, benefits, and working conditions, making it difficult to attract and retain skilled doctors, nurses, and other medical staff. As a result, there is an imbalance in the healthcare workforce, with an overwhelming workload burden on the existing healthcare professionals, leading to burnout and decreased quality of care.

3. Insufficient Infrastructure: Insufficient funding hinders the development and maintenance of healthcare infrastructure in Iran. Hospitals, clinics, and healthcare facilities struggle to upgrade and expand their infrastructure to meet the growing demands of the population. As a result, overcrowding, long waiting times, and inadequate facilities become common issues, compromising the overall patient experience and healthcare outcomes.

4. Limited Research and Development: Inadequate funding also impacts the investment in research and development within the healthcare sector. Lack of funding for medical research and innovation prevents the advancement of new treatments, technologies, and medical breakthroughs. This stagnation hampers the progress of medical science and limits the availability of cutting-edge treatments and therapies for patients in Iran.

Overall, inadequate funding severely hampers the delivery of healthcare services in Iran, leading to compromised patient care, limited access to essential medical equipment and supplies, a shortage of healthcare professionals, insufficient infrastructure, and a lack of progress in medical research and development. Addressing the funding gap is essential to improve the healthcare system and ensure better health outcomes for the Iranian population.

Inadequate funding directly affects the availability of medical equipment and supplies in healthcare facilities in several ways:

1. Limited Purchasing Power: Insufficient funds restrict the purchasing power of healthcare facilities. They are unable to afford the necessary medical equipment and supplies required to provide quality healthcare services. This includes diagnostic tools, surgical instruments, monitoring devices, and other essential medical devices. Without adequate funding, healthcare facilities cannot keep up with the demand for updated and modern equipment, which can directly impact patient care.

2. Outdated and Inefficient Equipment: Inadequate funding often leads to the continued use of outdated and inefficient medical equipment. Healthcare facilities may not have the resources to upgrade or replace old equipment, which can compromise the accuracy and

effectiveness of diagnoses and treatments. Outdated equipment may also require frequent repairs, leading to additional costs and downtime.

3. Limited Availability of Supplies: Insufficient funding can result in a shortage of medical supplies in healthcare facilities. This includes items such as medications, bandages, surgical gloves, and disinfectants. Without an adequate supply of these essential items, healthcare providers may be forced to ration or prioritize their use, potentially compromising patient safety and quality of care.

4. Inadequate Maintenance and Repairs: Inadequate funding can make it challenging for healthcare facilities to maintain and repair their existing medical equipment. Regular maintenance is crucial to ensure the proper functioning and longevity of equipment. Without sufficient funds, healthcare facilities may delay or neglect necessary maintenance, leading to equipment breakdowns and reduced availability.

5. Dependency on Donations: In the face of inadequate funding, healthcare facilities may become reliant on donations from individuals or organizations to acquire medical equipment and supplies. While donations can be helpful, they are often inconsistent and may not fully meet the needs of the healthcare facility. This dependency on donations can result in an unpredictable and unreliable supply of essential equipment and supplies.

Overall, inadequate funding directly impacts the availability and quality of medical equipment and supplies in healthcare facilities. Without sufficient resources, healthcare facilities struggle to purchase, upgrade, maintain, and repair equipment, leading to a scarcity of essential supplies and outdated technology. This can have a detrimental effect on the delivery of healthcare services and patient outcomes.

Healthcare facilities face several challenges in maintaining and repairing their existing medical equipment due to inadequate funding:

1. Limited Budget: Inadequate funding means that healthcare facilities have limited financial resources allocated for equipment maintenance and repairs. This limited budget makes it challenging to address all the maintenance needs of the facility, resulting in a backlog of repairs and potential equipment failures.

2. High Costs: The costs associated with maintaining and repairing medical equipment can be significant. This includes the cost of replacement parts, specialized tools, technician fees, and training. Inadequate funding makes it difficult for healthcare facilities to afford these expenses, leading to delays or neglect of necessary repairs.

3. Lack of Skilled Technicians: Maintaining and repairing medical equipment requires specialized knowledge and skills. Inadequate funding may result in a shortage of trained technicians who can effectively diagnose and fix equipment issues. Without skilled technicians, healthcare facilities may rely on inexperienced staff or outsource repairs, both of which can be costly and time-consuming.

4. Limited Access to Spare Parts: Medical equipment often requires specific spare parts for repairs. Inadequate funding may restrict the ability of healthcare facilities to access and purchase these spare parts. This can result in delays in repairs or the use of substandard parts, which can compromise the effectiveness and safety of the equipment.

5. Aging Equipment: Inadequate funding often means healthcare facilities are unable to replace outdated or aging equipment. Older equipment may require more frequent repairs and maintenance due to wear and tear. The lack of funds to replace or upgrade equipment can result in a continuous cycle of breakdowns and repairs, leading to increased costs and reduced availability.

6. Downtime and Disruption of Services: When medical equipment breaks down or requires repairs, it can result in downtime and disrupt healthcare services. Inadequate funding may prolong the downtime as healthcare facilities struggle to allocate funds for repairs. This can impact patient care, delay diagnoses, and treatments, and lead to increased wait times for medical procedures.

7. Safety Concerns: Inadequate funding for maintenance and repairs can compromise the safety of both patients and healthcare providers. Malfunctioning or poorly maintained equipment can result in inaccurate diagnoses, ineffective treatments, and potential harm to patients. It can also put healthcare providers at risk of injury or accidents.

Overall, inadequate funding poses significant challenges for healthcare facilities in maintaining and repairing their existing medical equipment. Limited budgets, high costs, a lack of skilled technicians, limited access to spare parts, aging equipment, downtime, and safety concerns all contribute to the difficulties faced by healthcare facilities in ensuring the proper functioning and longevity of their medical equipment.

Rebuilding a failed healthcare system requires a comprehensive and multi-faceted approach. While there is no one-size-fits-all solution, here are some short-term remedies and procedures that can help initiate the rebuilding process:

1. Increase Funding: Allocate immediate additional funding to the healthcare system to address critical infrastructure needs, equipment upgrades, and staffing requirements. This can help alleviate immediate resource shortages and improve the quality of care.

2. Improve Access to Healthcare: Implement measures to improve access to healthcare services, especially for marginalized and underserved populations. This can include expanding healthcare facilities, mobile clinics, and telemedicine services in remote areas, reducing waiting times for appointments, and ensuring affordable healthcare options for all.

3. Strengthen Primary Care: Focus on strengthening primary care services to ensure early detection, prevention, and management of diseases. This involves increasing the number of primary care providers, improving their training and resources, and promoting community-based healthcare initiatives.

4. Enhance Healthcare Workforce: Invest in the recruitment, training, and retention of healthcare professionals, including doctors, nurses, technicians, and support staff. Offer incentives and competitive salaries to attract skilled professionals and provide opportunities for ongoing professional development.

5. Implement Health Information Systems: Establish or improve health information systems to enable efficient data collection, analysis, and monitoring of healthcare services. This can help identify gaps, track patient outcomes, and facilitate evidence-based decision-making.

6. Strengthen Regulatory Framework: Enhance and enforce regulations to ensure quality standards, patient safety, and accountability in healthcare delivery. This includes regular inspections of healthcare facilities, monitoring of medical practices, and enforcement of ethical guidelines.

7. Collaborate with International Partners: Seek assistance and collaborate with international organizations, governments, and NGOs to access expertise, resources, and financial support. This can help in capacity building, knowledge sharing, and implementing best practices from successful healthcare systems.

8. Public Awareness and Education: Launch public awareness campaigns to educate the population about preventive healthcare measures, disease management, and available healthcare services. This can empower individuals to take responsibility for their health and reduce the burden on the healthcare system.

9. Prioritize Emergency Preparedness: Develop and implement robust emergency preparedness plans to handle public health crises effectively. This includes establishing protocols for rapid response, coordinating with relevant stakeholders, and ensuring adequate medical supplies and equipment.

10. Monitor and Evaluate Progress: Regularly monitor and evaluate the progress of healthcare system rebuilding efforts. Use data and feedback from patients, healthcare providers, and other stakeholders to identify areas of improvement and make necessary adjustments.

It is important to note that rebuilding a failed healthcare system is a complex and long-term process that requires sustained commitment, collaboration, and continuous evaluation. These short-term remedies and procedures can serve as a starting point for initiating the rebuilding process and laying the foundation for long-term sustainable healthcare reforms.

Improving access to healthcare services for marginalized and underserved populations requires targeted efforts and a comprehensive approach. Here are some strategies that can be implemented:

1. Increase Healthcare Facilities: Build or expand healthcare facilities in underserved areas, including rural and remote regions. This can include the establishment of community health

centers, mobile clinics, and telemedicine services to reach those who have limited access to traditional healthcare settings.

2. Improve Transportation: Address transportation barriers by providing affordable transportation options or arranging medical transportation services for individuals who have difficulty accessing healthcare facilities due to distance or lack of transportation.

3. Outreach Programs: Conduct targeted outreach programs to raise awareness about available healthcare services and resources. This can involve community-based initiatives, health fairs, and partnerships with local organizations to reach marginalized populations and provide them with information about healthcare options.

4. Culturally Competent Care: Train healthcare providers to deliver culturally competent care to diverse populations. This involves understanding and respecting cultural beliefs, practices, and language preferences, which can help build trust and improve patient-provider communication.

5. Language Services: Ensure language access by providing interpretation and translation services in healthcare settings. This can help individuals with limited English proficiency to communicate effectively with healthcare providers and understand their medical conditions and treatment options.

6. Financial Assistance: Implement programs and policies to make healthcare services more affordable for marginalized populations. This can include subsidies, sliding-scale payment options, and eligibility for government-funded healthcare programs.

7. Health Education: Promote health education and literacy among marginalized populations to empower individuals to take control of their health. This can involve providing information on preventive measures, disease management, and available healthcare resources through community workshops, educational materials, and digital platforms.

8. Community Health Workers: Train and deploy community health workers from within marginalized communities. These individuals can act as liaisons between the community and healthcare providers, offering culturally appropriate guidance, advocacy, and support in navigating the healthcare system.

9. Partnerships and Collaborations: Forge partnerships with community organizations, non-profit groups, and faith-based organizations to leverage their resources, networks, and expertise in reaching underserved populations. Collaborative efforts can help identify barriers and develop tailored solutions.

10. Data Collection and Analysis: Collect and analyze data on health disparities and access to healthcare services among marginalized populations. This can help identify gaps, measure progress, and inform evidence-based interventions to improve access and health outcomes.

It is essential to involve the affected communities in the planning and implementation of these strategies to ensure their needs and perspectives are considered. Additionally, ongoing evaluation and adjustment of these initiatives are crucial to address evolving challenges and ensure sustained improvement in access to healthcare services for marginalized and underserved populations.

Here are some strategies that can be implemented to improve access to healthcare services for marginalized and underserved populations:

1. Increase Healthcare Facilities: Build or expand healthcare facilities in underserved areas, including rural and remote regions. This can include the establishment of community health centers, mobile clinics, and telemedicine services to reach those who have limited access to traditional healthcare settings.

2. Improve Transportation: Address transportation barriers by providing affordable transportation options or arranging medical transportation services for individuals who have difficulty accessing healthcare facilities due to distance or lack of transportation.

3. Outreach Programs: Conduct targeted outreach programs to raise awareness about available healthcare services and resources. This can involve community-based initiatives, health fairs, and partnerships with local organizations to reach marginalized populations and provide them with information about healthcare options.

4. Culturally Competent Care: Train healthcare providers to deliver culturally competent care to diverse populations. This involves understanding and respecting cultural beliefs, practices, and language preferences, which can help build trust and improve patient-provider communication.

5. Language Services: Ensure language access by providing interpretation and translation services in healthcare settings. This can help individuals with limited English proficiency to communicate effectively with healthcare providers and understand their medical conditions and treatment options.

6. Financial Assistance: Implement programs and policies to make healthcare services more affordable for marginalized populations. This can include subsidies, sliding-scale payment options, and eligibility for government-funded healthcare programs.

7. Health Education: Promote health education and literacy among marginalized populations to empower individuals to take control of their health. This can involve providing information on preventive measures, disease management, and available healthcare resources through community workshops, educational materials, and digital platforms.

8. Community Health Workers: Train and deploy community health workers from within marginalized communities. These individuals can act as liaisons between the community and healthcare providers, offering culturally appropriate guidance, advocacy, and support

in navigating the healthcare system. Partnerships and Collaborations: Forge partnerships with community organizations, non-profit groups, and faith-based organizations to leverage their resources, networks, and expertise in reaching underserved populations. Collaborative efforts can help identify barriers and develop tailored solutions.

9. Data Collection and Analysis: Collect and analyze data on health disparities and access to healthcare services among marginalized populations. This can help identify gaps, measure progress, and inform evidence-based interventions to improve access and health outcomes.

By implementing these strategies, it is possible to address the barriers that marginalized and underserved populations face in accessing healthcare services and work towards achieving health equity for all.

Partnerships and collaborations with community organizations can play a vital role in reaching underserved populations in the following ways:

1. Trust and Credibility: Community organizations often have established trust and credibility within the communities they serve. Partnering with these organizations can help build trust and rapport with underserved populations, making it easier to engage and provide healthcare services.

2. Cultural Understanding: Community organizations have a deep understanding of the cultural norms, values, and beliefs of the population they serve. By collaborating with them, healthcare providers can gain insights into the unique needs and preferences of the community, ensuring that healthcare services are culturally appropriate and respectful.

3. Outreach and Awareness: Community organizations have existing networks and channels of communication to reach underserved populations. They can assist in conducting outreach activities, such as organizing health fairs, community workshops, and awareness campaigns, to educate the community about available healthcare services and resources.

4. Access Points: Community organizations often serve as access points for underserved populations. By partnering with these organizations, healthcare providers can leverage their existing infrastructure and resources to deliver healthcare services directly to the community. This can include setting up clinics or providing healthcare services within the organization's premises.

5. Navigating the System: Community organizations can help navigate the complex healthcare system on behalf of underserved populations. They can assist individuals in understanding eligibility criteria, completing paperwork, and accessing financial assistance programs or health insurance options.

6. Language and Cultural Mediation: Many community organizations have bilingual staff or volunteers who can act as interpreters and cultural mediators. This can facilitate effective

communication between healthcare providers and individuals with limited English proficiency, ensuring that they receive appropriate care and understand their treatment plans.

7. Tailored Interventions: Collaborating with community organizations allows healthcare providers to develop targeted interventions that address the specific needs and challenges faced by underserved populations. By working together, they can design and implement programs that are culturally sensitive, linguistically appropriate, and responsive to the community's unique circumstances.

8. Sustainability and Long-Term Impact: Partnerships with community organizations can contribute to sustainability and long-term impact. By involving the community in the planning and implementation of healthcare initiatives, there is a higher likelihood of acceptance, ownership, and continued engagement beyond the duration of the partnership.

Overall, partnerships and collaborations with community organizations provide a valuable opportunity to bridge the gap in healthcare access for underserved populations. By combining resources, expertise, and community knowledge, healthcare providers can effectively reach and serve those who might otherwise face barriers to accessing healthcare services.

Eliminating state-sponsored corruption in the healthcare system requires a multi-faceted approach that addresses the root causes and implements effective strategies. Here are some strategies that can help in combating corruption in the healthcare system:

1. Transparency and Accountability: Implementing transparent and accountable systems is crucial to prevent corruption. This can include establishing clear guidelines and procedures for procurement, financial management, and personnel appointments. Regular audits and independent oversight mechanisms should be put in place to ensure compliance and identify any irregularities.

2. Strengthening Legal and Regulatory Frameworks: Enact and enforce strong laws and regulations that explicitly address corruption in the healthcare sector. This includes criminalizing corrupt practices, ensuring protection for whistleblowers, and establishing effective mechanisms for reporting and investigating corruption cases. The penalties for corruption should be severe and enforced consistently.

3. Education and Training: Provide comprehensive training programs for healthcare professionals, administrators, and staff on ethics, integrity, and anti-corruption measures. This can help raise awareness about the negative impact of corruption, promote ethical behavior, and empower individuals to resist and report corrupt practices.

4. Encouraging Whistleblowing: Create a supportive environment for whistleblowers to come forward and report corruption without fear of retaliation. Establish confidential reporting mechanisms, protect the identity of whistleblowers, and ensure that appropriate

actions are taken to investigate and address reported cases. Strengthening Procurement Processes: Corruption often occurs during the procurement of medical supplies, equipment, and services. Implement robust procurement procedures that are transparent, competitive, and based on clear criteria. This can include open bidding, prequalification of suppliers, and regular monitoring of procurement processes to detect and prevent corrupt practices.

5. Technology and Digital Solutions: Utilize technology and digital solutions to minimize human intervention and reduce opportunities for corruption. Implement electronic medical records, e-procurement systems, and online payment mechanisms to enhance transparency, traceability, and efficiency in healthcare service delivery.

6. Public Awareness and Participation: Engage the public in the fight against corruption by raising awareness about the negative consequences of corruption in the healthcare system. Encourage active citizen participation through campaigns, advocacy, and the establishment of citizen oversight committees to monitor healthcare services and report any suspected corruption.

7. International Cooperation: Collaborate with international organizations, such as the World Health Organization (WHO) and United Nations Development Programme (UNDP), to access expertise, resources, and best practices in combating corruption in the healthcare sector. International cooperation can also help in strengthening governance frameworks and implementing anti-corruption measures.

8. Strong Leadership and Political Will: Effective leadership and political will are essential to drive anti-corruption efforts in the healthcare sector. Leaders should prioritize and demonstrate a zero-tolerance approach towards corruption, ensuring that appropriate resources and support are allocated to anti-corruption initiatives.

9. Strengthening Civil Society and Media: Support civil society organizations and media outlets to play an active role in exposing and combating corruption in the healthcare system. Provide platforms for public debate, investigative journalism, and civil society engagement to hold authorities accountable and advocate for transparency and integrity.

It is important to recognize that combating corruption is a long-term and ongoing process. Continuous monitoring, evaluation, and adaptation of strategies are necessary to ensure the effectiveness of anti-corruption measures in the healthcare system.

Some strategies that can help combat corruption in the healthcare system include:

1. Strengthening Legal and Regulatory Frameworks: Implement and enforce robust laws and regulations that explicitly address corruption in the healthcare sector. This includes criminalizing corrupt practices, establishing clear guidelines for procurement and financial management, and ensuring independent oversight and enforcement mechanisms.

2. Promoting Transparency and Accountability: Enhance transparency in healthcare systems by publishing information related to budgets, expenditures, and service delivery.

Implement mechanisms for public scrutiny and participation in decision-making processes. Hold healthcare providers and administrators accountable for their actions and establish effective mechanisms for reporting and investigating corruption cases.

3. Educating and Empowering Healthcare Professionals: Provide comprehensive training programs on ethics, integrity, and anti-corruption measures to healthcare professionals, administrators, and staff. Raise awareness about the negative impact of corruption and empower individuals to resist and report corrupt practices.

4. Strengthening Procurement Processes: Implement transparent and competitive procurement processes that are based on clear criteria and involve multiple stakeholders. Establish mechanisms to prevent conflicts of interest and ensure fair evaluation and selection of suppliers. Regularly monitor procurement processes to detect and prevent corrupt practices.

5. Encouraging Whistleblowing and Protecting Whistleblowers: Establish confidential reporting mechanisms and protection measures for whistleblowers. Encourage individuals to come forward with information about corruption and ensure that appropriate actions are taken to investigate and address reported cases. Protect whistleblowers from retaliation.

6. Utilizing Technology and Digital Solutions: Implement technology-driven solutions to minimize human intervention and reduce opportunities for corruption. This can include the use of e-procurement systems, electronic medical records, and online payment mechanisms that enhance transparency, traceability, and efficiency in healthcare service delivery.

7. Strengthening Internal Controls and Auditing Systems: Implement internal control mechanisms, such as regular audits, to detect and prevent corruption. Ensure that audits are conducted independently and that the findings are acted upon promptly. Implement effective risk management systems to identify and mitigate corruption risks.

8. Promoting Collaboration and International Cooperation: Collaborate with international organizations, governments, and civil society to share best practices, expertise, and resources in combating corruption in the healthcare sector. Engage in international initiatives and adopt international standards and guidelines for anti-corruption measures.

9. Fostering a Culture of Integrity and Ethics: Promote a culture of integrity and ethics within the healthcare system through codes of conduct, ethics committees, and training programs. Encourage leaders to lead by example and create an environment where ethical behavior is valued and rewarded.

10. Engaging Civil Society and Media: Encourage civil society organizations and media outlets to play an active role in monitoring and exposing corruption in the healthcare system. Support investigative journalism and advocacy efforts that raise awareness and hold authorities accountable.

It is important to recognize that combating corruption requires a comprehensive and multi-dimensional approach. These strategies should be implemented in a coordinated manner, with continuous monitoring, evaluation, and adaptation to ensure their effectiveness in combating corruption in the healthcare system.

Transparency and accountability in healthcare systems can be promoted through various strategies and measures. Here are some key approaches:

1. Publish Information: Healthcare systems should proactively publish information related to budgets, expenditures, healthcare outcomes, and service delivery. This includes making information accessible to the public through websites, reports, and other communication channels. By providing transparent information, stakeholders can better understand how resources are allocated and used in the healthcare system.

2. Enhance Financial Management: Implement robust financial management systems that promote accountability and transparency. This includes clear guidelines for budgeting, procurement, and financial reporting. Regular audits should be conducted to ensure compliance with financial regulations and identify any discrepancies or potential corruption.

3. Establish Oversight Mechanisms: Create independent oversight bodies or regulatory agencies responsible for monitoring and evaluating the performance of healthcare providers and administrators. These bodies should have the authority to investigate allegations of corruption and hold individuals accountable for their actions. They should also have the power to enforce sanctions and penalties when corruption is proven.

4. Strengthen Whistleblower Protection: Establish mechanisms to protect whistleblowers who report corruption in the healthcare system. This includes guaranteeing confidentiality, providing legal protection against retaliation, and offering incentives for reporting corruption. Whistleblower hotlines or online platforms can be set up to facilitate reporting and ensure anonymity.

5. Encourage Citizen Participation: Engage citizens in decision-making processes and allow them to provide feedback on healthcare services. This can be done through public consultations, citizen advisory committees, or patient satisfaction surveys. By involving the public, healthcare systems can ensure that decisions are made in the best interest of the population and hold providers accountable for their performance.

6. Implement Codes of Conduct and Ethics: Develop and enforce codes of conduct and ethics for healthcare professionals, administrators, and staff. These codes should clearly outline expected behaviors, ethical principles, and consequences for non-compliance. Regular ethics training programs can also be conducted to promote a culture of integrity and ethical decision-making.

7. Use Technology for Transparency: Leverage technology solutions to enhance transparency in healthcare systems. This can include the use of electronic medical records, online portals for accessing health information, and digital platforms for reporting and

tracking corruption cases. Technology can also streamline administrative processes, reducing the opportunities for corruption.

8. Conduct Independent Evaluations and Audits: Regularly evaluate the performance and effectiveness of healthcare systems through independent evaluations and audits. These assessments should be conducted by external experts or agencies to ensure objectivity and impartiality. The findings should be made public, and actions should be taken to address any identified weaknesses or corruption risks.

9. Foster Collaboration and Partnerships: Foster collaboration between government agencies, civil society organizations, and other stakeholders to promote transparency and accountability in healthcare systems. This can involve sharing best practices, exchanging information, and coordinating efforts to address corruption. International cooperation and partnerships can also provide valuable insights and support in combating corruption.

10. Promote Media and Civil Society Engagement: Encourage media outlets and civil society organizations to actively monitor and investigate corruption in the healthcare system. Support investigative journalism and advocacy efforts that expose corruption cases and hold authorities accountable. This can create public awareness and pressure for reform.

It is crucial to ensure that these strategies are implemented in a comprehensive and coordinated manner, with continuous monitoring and evaluation to assess their effectiveness. By promoting transparency and accountability, healthcare systems can improve trust, efficiency, and the quality of care provided to the population.

Technology solutions can play a significant role in enhancing transparency in healthcare systems. Here are some ways technology can be used to promote transparency:

1. Electronic Health Records (EHRs): Electronic health records digitize patient information, making it easily accessible and shareable among healthcare providers. This improves transparency by allowing authorized healthcare professionals to access a patient's medical history, test results, and treatment plans. It reduces errors, and duplication of tests, and improves coordination of care across different healthcare settings.

2. Health Information Exchange (HIE): Health information exchange platforms facilitate the secure sharing of patient data among different healthcare organizations. By enabling the seamless transfer of information, HIEs promote transparency and enhance care coordination. They allow physicians to access vital patient information in real time, resulting in better-informed decisions and improved patient outcomes.

3. Telemedicine and Remote Monitoring: Telemedicine enables remote consultations and monitoring of patients, particularly useful in underserved areas or during emergencies. It enhances transparency by providing patients with increased access to healthcare services and medical expertise. Telemedicine also allows for remote monitoring of patient's vital

signs and health conditions, providing real-time data to healthcare providers for better decision-making.

4. Mobile Applications and Wearable Devices: Mobile applications and wearable devices enable individuals to monitor their health, track fitness, and manage chronic conditions. These technologies promote transparency by empowering patients to actively participate in their care. They can access their health information, track progress, and share data with healthcare providers, leading to more informed discussions and personalized care plans.

5. Data Analytics and Business Intelligence: Advanced data analytics and business intelligence tools can analyze large volumes of healthcare data to identify patterns, trends, and anomalies. These technologies enhance transparency by providing insights into healthcare outcomes, resource utilization, and cost-effectiveness. They enable healthcare organizations to make data-driven decisions, optimize operations, and identify areas for improvement.

6. Fraud Detection and Prevention: Technology solutions can be used to detect and prevent healthcare fraud and abuse. AI-powered algorithms can analyze healthcare claims data to identify irregularities and patterns indicative of fraudulent activities. These solutions help healthcare organizations and regulatory bodies in monitoring and investigating potential cases of fraud, promoting transparency and accountability in financial transactions.

7. Online Portals and Patient Engagement: Online portals provide patients with access to their health records, appointment scheduling, and educational resources. They promote transparency by enabling patients to actively engage in their care, review and verify their health information, and communicate securely with healthcare providers. Patient portals also enhance transparency by providing transparent pricing information and facilitating billing and insurance processes.

8. Blockchain Technology: Blockchain technology offers secure and transparent record-keeping of healthcare transactions and data exchanges. It ensures the integrity and immutability of data, reducing the risk of tampering or unauthorized access. Blockchain can be used for secure sharing of health records, tracking the supply chain of pharmaceuticals, and managing consent for data sharing, enhancing transparency and data security.

9. Open Data Initiatives: Governments and healthcare organizations can promote transparency by implementing open data initiatives. By making non-sensitive healthcare data publicly available in a standardized and machine-readable format, researchers, policymakers, and the public can access and analyze the data to gain insights and hold healthcare systems accountable.

10. Reporting and Feedback Systems: Technology can facilitate the implementation of reporting and feedback systems to collect patient feedback, complaints, and suggestions. Online platforms or mobile applications can allow patients to report adverse events, share their experiences, and rate healthcare services. These systems promote transparency by

providing a channel for patients to voice their concerns and contribute to quality improvement efforts.

By leveraging technology solutions, healthcare systems can enhance transparency, promote patient engagement, improve decision-making, and facilitate the delivery of quality and accountable care. However, it is essential to consider data privacy and security measures to protect sensitive health information and ensure the ethical use of technology in healthcare.

Electronic Health Records (EHRs) can significantly improve transparency in healthcare by enhancing access to patient information, promoting communication and collaboration among healthcare providers, and enabling better-informed decision-making. Here are some ways EHRs contribute to transparency:

1. Centralized and Accessible Patient Information: EHRs consolidate patient information into a single digital record, making it easily accessible to authorized healthcare providers. This eliminates the need for manual paper records and reduces the risk of data fragmentation. Having a centralized and comprehensive view of a patient's medical history, medications, allergies, and test results improves transparency by ensuring that healthcare providers have accurate and up-to-date information when making diagnoses and treatment decisions.

2. Care Coordination and Continuity: EHRs enable seamless sharing of patient information among different healthcare settings and providers. This promotes transparency by facilitating care coordination and continuity. When multiple healthcare providers are involved in a patient's care, EHRs allow them to access the same information, reducing the chances of errors, duplication of tests, and unnecessary procedures. It improves transparency by ensuring that all providers involved in a patient's care have access to the same information, leading to more coordinated and effective treatment plans.

3. Medication Management: EHRs include medication lists, drug interaction alerts, and allergy information, improving transparency in medication management. Healthcare providers can review a patient's medication history, including prescriptions, dosages, and refill information, promoting better-informed decisions and reducing the risk of medication errors. EHRs can also provide decision support tools, such as drug formularies and clinical guidelines, further enhancing transparency in medication prescribing and monitoring.

4. Patient Engagement: EHRs can empower patients to actively participate in their healthcare and improve transparency. Patient portals connected to EHRs allow individuals to access their health records, review test results, and communicate securely with healthcare providers. Patients can verify the accuracy of their health information, ask questions, and provide additional details about their medical history. This promotes transparency by fostering a collaborative relationship between patients and healthcare providers, where both parties have access to the same information and can make informed decisions together. Data Analytics and Population Health Management: EHRs generate

vast amounts of data that can be analyzed to identify trends, patterns, and outcomes at both the individual and population levels. By analyzing EHR data, healthcare organizations can gain insights into disease prevalence, treatment effectiveness, and resource utilization. This promotes transparency by enabling healthcare providers and policymakers to make data-driven decisions, identify areas for improvement, and measure the quality and efficiency of care provided.

5. Quality Reporting and Auditing: EHRs can facilitate quality reporting and auditing processes. With structured and standardized data captured in EHRs, healthcare organizations can generate reports on quality measures, compliance with clinical guidelines, and patient outcomes. These reports promote transparency by allowing healthcare providers to assess their performance, compare it to benchmarks, and identify areas for improvement. EHRs also facilitate auditing processes by providing a detailed audit trail of who accessed, modified, or shared patient information, enhancing transparency and accountability in data handling.

6. Research and Knowledge Sharing: EHRs can contribute to medical research and knowledge sharing. De-identified and aggregated EHR data can be used for research purposes, allowing researchers to study disease patterns, treatment effectiveness, and population health trends. EHRs also facilitate the sharing of best practices and clinical knowledge among healthcare providers, promoting transparency and collaboration in evidence-based medicine.

By leveraging the capabilities of EHR systems, healthcare organizations can enhance transparency, improve patient care, and drive better health outcomes. However, it is crucial to ensure proper privacy and security measures are in place to protect patient data and maintain trust in the system.

Electronic Health Records (EHRs) contribute to transparency in healthcare in several ways:

1. Improved Access to Information: EHRs provide healthcare providers with instant access to comprehensive patient information, including medical history, diagnoses, medications, allergies, and test results. This improves transparency by ensuring that healthcare providers have a complete and accurate picture of a patient's health, enabling better-informed decision-making.

2. Enhanced Communication and Collaboration: EHRs facilitate communication and collaboration among healthcare providers. Different providers involved in a patient's care can access and share information through the EHR system, promoting transparency by ensuring that all relevant parties have access to the same information. This leads to more coordinated and integrated care, reducing errors and improving patient outcomes.

3. Patient Involvement: EHRs allow patients to access their health information through secure patient portals. Patients can review their medical records, test results, and treatment

plans, promoting transparency by empowering them to actively participate in their healthcare decisions. Patients can also provide additional information and correct any inaccuracies, ensuring that the EHR reflects their complete medical history.

4. Medication Safety: EHRs include medication lists, drug interaction alerts, and allergy information. Healthcare providers can access a patient's medication history, reducing the risk of medication errors, adverse drug reactions, and duplicate prescriptions. This promotes transparency in medication management, ensuring that healthcare providers have accurate and up-to-date information to make safe prescribing decisions.

5. Decision Support: EHRs often include decision support tools such as clinical guidelines, drug formularies, and alerts for potential drug interactions or allergies. These tools assist healthcare providers in making evidence-based decisions, improving transparency by providing access to the latest medical knowledge and best practices.

6. Data Analytics and Reporting: EHRs generate vast amounts of data that can be analyzed to identify trends, patterns, and outcomes. Healthcare organizations can analyze this data to measure and report on quality indicators, population health trends, and healthcare outcomes. This promotes transparency by allowing healthcare providers and policymakers to assess performance, identify areas for improvement, and make data-driven decisions.

7. Privacy and Security: EHRs have built-in privacy and security measures to protect patient information. Access to patient records is regulated, and audit trails track who accessed, modified, or shared patient data. These measures promote transparency by ensuring that patient information is securely handled, maintaining trust in the healthcare system.

8. Research and Population Health: EHRs can contribute to medical research and population health management. De-identified and aggregated EHR data can be used for research purposes, allowing researchers to study disease patterns, treatment effectiveness, and population health trends. This promotes transparency by facilitating knowledge-sharing and advancing evidence-based medicine.

By leveraging the capabilities of EHR systems, healthcare organizations can improve transparency, enhance patient care, and drive better health outcomes. However, it is essential to address privacy concerns and ensure that proper safeguards are in place to protect patient confidentiality and data security.

Combating fraud in medical education within a failed system can be challenging, but several strategies can be implemented to address the issue:

1. Strengthen Regulatory Oversight: Enhance regulatory oversight and enforcement to ensure compliance with standards and regulations. This includes monitoring the accreditation process, conducting regular inspections, and implementing strict penalties for institutions found involved in fraudulent activities.

2. Improve Transparency and Accountability: Increase transparency in the medical education system by providing clear and accessible information about institutions, programs, faculty, and accreditation status. Establish mechanisms for reporting and addressing fraudulent activities, such as anonymous reporting hotlines or whistleblower protection programs.

3. Implement Accreditation Reforms: Enhance the accreditation process by implementing stricter criteria and evaluation methods. This could include more frequent and thorough site visits, evaluation of faculty qualifications, and student outcomes assessment. Accrediting bodies should also be independent and have the necessary resources and authority to enforce standards effectively.

4. Strengthen Collaboration and Information Sharing: Foster collaboration among regulatory bodies, medical associations, and educational institutions to share information and best practices for detecting and preventing fraud. Establish mechanisms for sharing information about fraudulent institutions or individuals to ensure that they are not able to operate across different jurisdictions.

5. Enhance Professionalism and Ethics Education: Incorporate a strong emphasis on professionalism, ethics, and integrity within medical education curricula. Teach students about the consequences of fraud, the importance of honesty, and the ethical responsibilities associated with being a healthcare professional.

6. Implement Financial Controls: Implement financial controls and audits to detect and prevent fraudulent financial practices. This could include regular audits of institutional finances, ensuring proper use of tuition fees, and increasing financial transparency.

7. Encourage Whistleblowing and Protection: Create a culture that encourages whistleblowing by providing protection and incentives for individuals who report fraudulent activities. Establish mechanisms to investigate and address reports promptly and confidentially.

8. Engage Stakeholders: Involve stakeholders, including students, faculty, medical associations, and regulatory bodies, in the decision-making process to address fraud in medical education. Their input and involvement can help identify potential issues and develop effective solutions.

9. Strengthen International Cooperation: Collaborate with international organizations and regulatory bodies to address fraud in medical education that may cross national borders. Share information, harmonize standards, and collaborate on enforcement efforts to prevent fraudulent institutions from operating globally.

10. Continuous Monitoring and Evaluation: Regularly monitor and evaluate the effectiveness of implemented measures to combat fraud in medical education. Adjust and improve strategies as needed to stay ahead of fraudulent practices and adapt to changing circumstances.

Addressing fraud in medical education requires a multi-faceted approach involving strong regulatory oversight, collaboration among stakeholders, and a commitment to professionalism and integrity. It is essential to create a system that promotes transparency, accountability, and ethical conduct to ensure the quality and integrity of medical education.

To enhance regulatory oversight and enforcement in combating fraud in medical education, here are some strategies that can be implemented:

1. Strengthen Regulatory Framework: Review and revise the existing regulatory framework to ensure it is comprehensive, up-to-date, and aligned with international standards. This may involve updating laws, regulations, and guidelines to address emerging issues and challenges related to fraud in medical education.

2. Increase Resources and Expertise: Allocate sufficient resources, both financial and human, to regulatory bodies responsible for overseeing medical education. This includes hiring qualified staff with expertise in fraud detection and investigation, as well as providing them with the necessary training and tools to effectively carry out their responsibilities.

3. Conduct Regular Inspections and Audits: Implement a system of regular inspections and audits of medical institutions to assess their compliance with regulatory standards and identify any signs of fraudulent activities. Inspections should be thorough, unannounced, and cover all aspects of the educational institution, including faculty qualifications, curriculum, facilities, and financial records.

4. Strengthen Collaboration with Law Enforcement: Foster collaboration and information sharing between regulatory bodies and law enforcement agencies. Establish formal channels of communication and coordination to facilitate the investigation and prosecution of fraudulent activities in medical education. This may involve creating joint task forces or working groups dedicated to combating fraud in the sector.

5. Implement Whistleblower Protection Mechanisms: Establish mechanisms to protect and incentivize whistleblowers who come forward with information about fraudulent practices in medical education. Ensure that individuals who report fraud are protected from retaliation and that their identities are kept confidential. Provide appropriate incentives, such as monetary rewards or legal protections, to encourage reporting.

6. Implement Risk-Based Approaches: Adopt risk-based approaches to prioritize oversight efforts and allocate resources effectively. Identify high-risk areas or institutions based on factors such as past violations, student complaints, financial irregularities, or accreditation status. Focus regulatory efforts on these high-risk areas to maximize the impact of oversight and enforcement activities.

7. Enhance Data Collection and Analysis: Improve data collection and analysis systems to identify patterns and trends related to fraud in medical education. Utilize technology and data analytics to monitor key indicators, such as student outcomes, graduation rates, and

financial transactions, to detect potentially fraudulent activities. Regularly analyze data to identify outliers or anomalies that may indicate fraudulent practices.

8. Strengthen Accreditation Processes: Collaborate with accrediting bodies to strengthen the accreditation process and ensure that it includes robust measures for fraud detection and prevention. This may involve enhancing the criteria for accreditation, conducting more frequent and thorough site visits, and ensuring that accreditation bodies have the necessary resources and authority to enforce standards effectively.

9. Encourage Reporting and Complaint Mechanisms: Establish clear reporting and complaint mechanisms for students, faculty, and other stakeholders to report suspected fraudulent activities. Ensure that these mechanisms are easily accessible, confidential, and well-publicized. Provide appropriate channels for individuals to report anonymously if they prefer.

10. Implement Strict Penalties and Enforcement Actions: Enforce strict penalties and take decisive enforcement actions against institutions found involved in fraudulent practices. This may include revoking accreditation, imposing fines, suspending or revoking licenses, and pursuing legal action against individuals or institutions engaged in fraudulent activities. Ensure that enforcement actions are publicized to serve as a deterrent to others.

By implementing these strategies, regulatory bodies can enhance their oversight and enforcement efforts to combat fraud in medical education effectively. It is crucial to adopt a proactive and collaborative approach involving all stakeholders to maintain the integrity and quality of medical education.

During regular inspections and audits of medical institutions, several key aspects should be covered to identify signs of fraudulent activities. These aspects include:

1. Faculty Qualifications: Verify the qualifications and credentials of the faculty members. Ensure that they have the necessary education, training, and experience to teach the courses they are assigned to. Look for any discrepancies or false claims regarding their qualifications.

2. Curriculum and Course Offerings: Review the curriculum and course offerings to ensure they meet the required standards and are aligned with the stated objectives of the medical education program. Check for any irregularities, such as courses that are not relevant to the program or courses that are not being taught as required.

3. Student Admissions and Enrollment: Examine the process of student admissions and enrollment to ensure it is fair, transparent, and based on merit. Look for any signs of preferential treatment or manipulation of admissions criteria. Check if the number of enrolled students matches the reported figures and if there are any discrepancies.

4. Student Progress and Assessment: Assess the mechanisms in place to monitor student progress and evaluate their performance. Look for any signs of grade inflation or manipulation of assessment results. Ensure that students are being adequately assessed and

that their progress is being accurately recorded. Facilities and Resources: Inspect the facilities and resources available to students, including classrooms, laboratories, libraries, and clinical facilities. Check if they meet the required standards and are appropriate for delivering quality medical education. Look for any signs of inadequate resources or misrepresentation of facilities.

5. Financial Management: Scrutinize the financial records and management practices of the institution. Verify the accuracy and transparency of financial transactions, including tuition fees, scholarships, and other revenue sources. Look for any signs of financial irregularities, such as embezzlement, money laundering, or misappropriation of funds.

6. Student Support Services: Evaluate the availability and effectiveness of student support services, including counseling, career guidance, and academic support. Ensure that students are receiving the necessary support to succeed in their medical education. Look for any signs of inadequate support services or false claims regarding the availability of these services.

7. Compliance with Regulatory Standards: Assess the institution's compliance with regulatory standards and guidelines. Verify if the institution has obtained the necessary licenses, accreditations, and certifications required for operating a medical education program. Look for any violations or non-compliance with regulatory requirements.

8. Stakeholder Feedback: Gather feedback from students, faculty, and other stakeholders about their experiences with the institution. Conduct interviews or surveys to assess the satisfaction levels and identify any concerns or complaints. Look for any consistent patterns or recurring issues raised by stakeholders.

9. Documentation and Record-Keeping: Review the institution's documentation and record-keeping practices. Ensure that all relevant records, such as student records, faculty qualifications, financial statements, and accreditation documents, are maintained accurately and are easily accessible. Look for any signs of tampering or falsification of records.

By thoroughly examining these key aspects during inspections and audits, regulatory bodies can identify potential signs of fraudulent activities in medical institutions. It is essential to have trained auditors or inspectors who are knowledgeable about fraud detection techniques and can effectively identify red flags or indicators of fraudulent practices.

During inspections and audits of medical institutions, several key aspects should be covered to ensure compliance, quality, and patient safety. These aspects include:

1. Regulatory Compliance: Assess the institution's compliance with applicable laws, regulations, and standards set by regulatory bodies. This includes verifying licenses, permits, certifications, and adherence to guidelines related to healthcare, patient care, safety, and privacy.

2. Facility and Equipment: Inspect the physical facilities, infrastructure, and equipment used for patient care, diagnosis, treatment, and research. Ensure that they meet safety standards, are properly maintained, and are suitable for their intended purposes.

3. Medical Records and Documentation: Review the completeness, accuracy, and confidentiality of medical records and documentation. Assess if records are properly maintained, easily accessible, and contain relevant information required for patient care, billing, and legal purposes.

4. Quality Assurance and Improvement: Evaluate the institution's quality assurance and improvement programs. This includes monitoring and evaluating the quality of care, patient outcomes, infection control measures, medication management, and compliance with clinical protocols.

5. Human Resources: Assess the qualifications, training, and competence of healthcare professionals, including physicians, nurses, technicians, and support staff. Verify credentials, licenses, certifications, and adherence to professional standards and code of ethics.

6. Patient Safety and Care: Evaluate the institution's policies, procedures, and practices related to patient safety, infection control, medication safety, and adverse event reporting. Ensure that systems are in place to identify, prevent, and respond to patient safety incidents.

7. Financial Management: Scrutinize financial practices, including billing, coding, reimbursement, and financial controls. Verify the accuracy and transparency of financial transactions, adherence to billing regulations, and prevention of fraud, waste, and abuse.

8. Research and Ethics: Assess the institution's research activities, including compliance with ethical standards, protection of research participants, and proper documentation of research protocols and findings.

9. Information Technology and Data Security: Evaluate the institution's information technology systems, electronic health records, and data security measures. Verify the protection of patient information, data integrity, and compliance with privacy regulations.

10. Stakeholder Feedback: Gather feedback from patients, staff, and other stakeholders about their experiences with the institution. This feedback can help identify areas for improvement, patient satisfaction levels, and any concerns or complaints.

By covering these key aspects during inspections and audits, regulatory bodies, accreditation agencies, and quality improvement organizations can ensure that medical institutions meet the required standards, provide quality care, and maintain patient safety. Additionally, these assessments help identify areas for improvement and support continuous quality enhancement in healthcare delivery.

Gathering feedback from patients, staff, and other stakeholders during inspections and audits of medical institutions is important for several reasons:

1. Patient-Centered Care: Patient feedback provides valuable insights into the quality of care and services provided by the medical institution. It helps assess whether the institution is meeting patient needs, expectations, and preferences. Gathering patient feedback ensures that the institution is delivering patient-centered care and can identify areas for improvement.

2. Quality Improvement: Feedback from patients and staff can pinpoint areas that require improvement in the institution's processes, policies, and practices. It provides an opportunity to identify gaps in care, potential risks, and areas where patient safety can be enhanced. By incorporating feedback into quality improvement initiatives, medical institutions can enhance the overall quality of care they provide.

3. Staff Engagement and Satisfaction: Staff feedback is crucial for assessing their engagement, satisfaction, and well-being. It allows the institution to understand the concerns and challenges faced by staff members, which can impact their performance and the quality of care provided. Addressing staff concerns and involving them in decision-making processes can improve morale, teamwork, and overall performance.

4. Stakeholder Perspectives: Gathering feedback from other stakeholders, such as referring physicians, community organizations, and regulatory bodies, provides a broader perspective on the institution's performance. It helps identify opportunities for collaboration and areas for improvement and ensures that the institution is meeting the expectations and requirements of various stakeholders.

5. Compliance and Accreditation: Regulatory bodies and accreditation agencies often require evidence of patient and stakeholder feedback as part of the compliance and accreditation process. Gathering feedback demonstrates the institution's commitment to continuous improvement, patient safety, and meeting regulatory standards.

6. Transparency and Accountability: By actively seeking feedback, medical institutions demonstrate transparency and accountability to their patients, staff, and stakeholders. It shows a willingness to listen, address concerns, and make necessary changes to enhance the quality of care.

7. Patient Satisfaction and Loyalty: Positive patient feedback can contribute to increased patient satisfaction and loyalty. Patients who feel heard and valued are more likely to have a positive perception of the institution and recommend it to others. This can lead to improved patient retention, increased referrals, and a positive reputation in the community.

In summary, gathering feedback from patients, staff, and other stakeholders during inspections and audits of medical institutions is essential for assessing the quality of care, identifying areas for improvement, enhancing patient safety, and ensuring compliance with regulatory standards. It promotes patient-centered care, staff engagement, and continuous quality improvement in healthcare delivery.

State of Chaos, Ideological Dogmatism, aftermath and hopes

In a world plagued by the grip of fascism and ideological dictatorship, the rights and freedoms of citizens are trampled upon, leaving a trail of devastation in its wake. The very essence of democracy is undermined as those in power prioritize their interests over the well-being of the people they are meant to serve.

Under such a regime, the systematic abuse of power becomes the norm. Citizens are subjected to surveillance, intimidation, and oppression, their voices silenced, and their autonomy stripped away. The government, driven by a twisted ideology, seeks to control every aspect of their lives, leaving no room for dissent or individuality.

Corruption, like a cancer, spreads throughout every level of the system. The once noble purpose of governance is perverted, as those in power exploit their positions for personal gain. Public resources are siphoned away, leaving the citizens in dire straits while a privileged few revel in their ill-gotten wealth. The very institutions that should protect and serve the people become tools of oppression and instruments of greed.

In this dystopian reality, basic human rights are denied with impunity. Freedom of speech, thought, and expression are curtailed, leaving citizens fearful of expressing their opinions or challenging the status quo. Dissidents are silenced, imprisoned, or worse, while the government creates a climate of fear and conformity.

Moreover, the denial of citizens' rights to healthcare, education, and freedom further exacerbates the suffering of the people. Healthcare, a fundamental human right, becomes a luxury accessible only to the elite, leaving the majority to suffer without access to proper medical care. Education, the key to a better future, is restricted and manipulated, depriving citizens of the knowledge and skills they need to thrive.

The denial of freedom, healthcare, and education is not only a violation of human rights but also a blatant disregard for the well-being and potential of the citizens. It perpetuates a cycle of inequality and injustice, reinforcing the power imbalance between the ruling class and the oppressed masses.

In the face of such tyranny, the international community must stand united against fascism and ideological dictatorship. Governments and organizations must come together to condemn these flagrant abuses, applying diplomatic and economic pressure to bring about change. Humanitarian aid should be provided to alleviate the suffering of the citizens, and efforts must be made to support grassroots movements that strive for freedom, justice, and equality.

The struggle against fascism and ideological dictatorship is an arduous one, but history has shown us that the power of unity, resilience, and the unwavering belief in the inherent rights and dignity of every individual can triumph over oppression. It is our collective responsibility to challenge and dismantle these oppressive systems, to restore the rights and freedoms that have been denied, and to create a world where every citizen can flourish without fear or discrimination.

Once upon a time in a country home to epic heroes' brave and noble characters, Iran was plagued by a failed and reactionary government, and the state of healthcare was dire. The system was fragmented, ineffective, and inaccessible to most of the population. People suffered, lives were lost, and hope seemed distant. But amidst this turmoil, a collective voice of change began to rise, fueled by the determination and resilience of the citizens.

In this country, I had the privilege of witnessing the power of unity and creativity as individuals came together to tackle the state of chaos and human rights crisis. Despite the challenges posed by the government's lack of vision, the people refused to be defeated. They understood that a healthy nation was the cornerstone of progress and happiness, and they were determined to bring about change.

In the face of a failing government, innovative grassroots movements emerged to bridge the gaps in the healthcare and education systems. Local communities organized underground health camps, where doctors and nurses volunteered their time and expertise to treat those in need and many lost their lives in the process These cliques became beacons of hope, offering free medical care, essential medicines, and health education to the underprivileged.

Furthermore, altruistic individuals formed networks to share resources and knowledge, creating a support system that extended beyond the limitations imposed by the government. They organized fundraisers, donated medical equipment, and established community health centers to ensure that healthcare was accessible to all, regardless of their social or economic status.

The power of technology also played a significant role in this healthcare revolution. Tech-savvy individuals used social media platforms to raise awareness about the dire situation, shedding light on the government's negligence and inspiring others to act. Online platforms were created to connect patients with doctors willing to offer telemedicine consultations, providing a lifeline to those in remote areas and underserved communities.

As the movement gained momentum, it caught the attention of many physicians, inside and abroad, and compassionate individuals globally. Medical professionals from around the world volunteered their time to travel to this country, providing specialized care and sharing their expertise with local doctors and nurses. Humanitarian aid poured in, helping to bolster the efforts of the people and alleviate the burden on the failing government, many of these individuals were detained, imprisoned and groups were deported, and medical cargo and equipment were confiscated.

In the face of adversity, the citizens of this country refused to let their government's failures define them. Their collective determination and resilience transformed the communities, their beliefs and political landscape. The movement for change, driven by compassion, creativity, and the unwavering belief in a brighter future, became a catalyst for reform.

Gradually, faced with mounting pressure, the government although confused and politically incoherent became more vicious with boots on the ground killing innocent citizens, refusing the grassroots movements, denying their innovative approaches, and incorporating them into their policies. The country was engulfed in chaos and horror, but the nation was hopeful and resilient.

Banners and slogans with defiance messages were placed across the country and steganography messages were distributed countrywide.

In time, the once-failed healthcare system became a source of pride for the nation. Access to quality care became a fundamental right, and no longer was healthcare a privilege reserved for the elite. The country's journey from despair to hope became an inspirational tale, reminding the world of the power of unity, creativity, and the resilience of the human spirit.

Throughout history, Iran has endured immense hardship, occupation, mass killings, and devastating destruction. However, it has consistently risen from the ashes, emerging more distinguished and advanced each time.

Iranians learned how the determination and ingenuity of individuals can overcome the challenges posed by a failed and reactionary government. By working together, embracing innovation, and refusing to give up, the citizens of this country transformed their lives and governing system and paved the way for a brighter future.

Monastic Medicine

In the quiet and serene lands of medieval Europe, nestled amongst lush green fields, stood a grand monastery. The monastery was not only a place of worship but also a sanctuary for those seeking solace and healing. Within its walls resided a group of dedicated monks, known for their knowledge and practice of monastic medicine.

The monks had devoted their lives to serving others, not only through prayer and spiritual guidance but also through their extensive knowledge of medicinal herbs and remedies. Passed down through generations, their wisdom in healing was deeply rooted in ancient texts and the teachings of renowned physicians of the time.

Brother Thomas, a kind-hearted monk with a gentle smile, was particularly known for his expertise in monastic medicine. With his long gray beard and a twinkle in his eyes, he possessed a wealth of knowledge about the healing properties of plants and the balance of the body's humor.

One summer day, a young traveler named James arrived at the monastery seeking help. He had been suffering from a mysterious ailment that caused him great pain and discomfort.

Hearing of Brother Thomas' reputation as a skilled healer, James sought his guidance in hopes of finding relief.

Brother Thomas welcomed James warmly, inviting him into the monastery's infirmary. The room was filled with the aroma of medicinal herbs, and shelves were lined with jars containing various potions and tinctures. Brother Thomas carefully examined James, listening attentively to his symptoms and asking detailed questions about his lifestyle and habits.

As the sun began to set, Brother Thomas prepared a soothing herbal tea for James, carefully selecting a blend of chamomile, lavender, and lemon balm known for their calming properties. He explained to James that relaxation and stress relief were essential in aiding the body's natural healing processes.

Days turned into weeks, and James remained under the watchful care of Brother Thomas. Each day, the monk administered various herbal remedies, prepared poultices, and even performed gentle massages to alleviate James' pain and promote his well-being. Additionally, Brother Thomas encouraged James to adopt a healthy lifestyle, emphasizing the importance of exercise, proper nutrition, and a balanced spiritual life.

With time, James started to experience a gradual improvement in his condition. His pain subsided, and he regained his strength and vitality. The young traveler was filled with gratitude for the monks and their unique approach to healing.

As James bid farewell to the monastery, he thanked Brother Thomas for his exceptional care and shared his newfound belief in the power of monastic medicine. He promised to spread the word of their healing practices to others in need, ensuring that the wisdom of the monks would reach far and wide.

And so, the legacy of monastic medicine continued to thrive, offering solace and healing to countless souls who sought the gentle touch of the monks' knowledge and compassion. Through their dedication and the power of nature's remedies, they brought hope and relief to those in need, leaving a lasting impression on the history of medicine.

Arab Medicine:

In the vast and arid lands of the Arab Peninsula, where the golden sun scorched the desert sands, a rich history of medicine emerged, intertwined with the vibrant tapestry of Arab culture and knowledge. For centuries, the people of the Arab Peninsula sought solace and healing through a unique blend of traditional practices, herbal remedies, and the wisdom of ancient scholars.

In the early days of Arab civilization, the nomadic Bedouin tribes relied on their deep connection with nature to heal their ailments. They had a profound understanding of the medicinal properties of plants and herbs that thrived in the harsh desert environment. From the soothing aloe vera to the aromatic frankincense, they harnessed the healing powers of these natural wonders.

As the Arab Peninsula became a crossroads of trade and cultural exchange, the knowledge of medicine began to flourish. The city of Mecca, with its bustling markets and diverse population, became a melting pot of ideas and practices from the East and the West. Arab physicians eagerly absorbed the wisdom of Indian, Persian, and Greek medicine, blending it with their traditional remedies.

One of the most prominent figures in the history of medicine in the Arab Peninsula was Ibn Sina, better known as Avicenna. Born in present-day Uzbekistan (Persia), Avicenna was a polymath whose contributions to medicine were revolutionary. His masterpiece, "The Canon of Medicine," became a seminal text that influenced medical practice for centuries to come.

Avicenna's work emphasized the importance of observation, diagnosis, and the holistic approach to medicine. He believed that the body and mind were interconnected, and health could only be achieved through a balance of the four humors - blood, phlegm, yellow bile, and black bile. His knowledge of pharmacology also led to the development of innovative herbal remedies and the establishment of pharmacies throughout the region.

The Arab Peninsula continued to be a hub of medical advancement as Islamic civilization flourished. The Abbasid Caliphate in Baghdad became a center of learning, attracting scholars, physicians, and translators from around the world. Persian physicians, such as Razi, and Muslim Spain physicians such as Al-Zahrawi, made remarkable contributions to medicine, exploring new surgical techniques, developing medical instruments, and compiling extensive encyclopedias of medical knowledge.

The rise of universities and libraries in major cities like Cairo, Damascus, and Cordoba further propelled the progress of medicine in the Arab Peninsula. These institutions became beacons of intellectual exchange, where scholars and students gathered to study and expand their understanding of the human body, diseases, and treatments.

Arab medicine also made significant strides in the field of ophthalmology. Pioneering surgeons like Al-Mawsili and Ibn Al-Haytham perfected techniques for cataract surgery and devised innovative tools for eye examinations. Their contributions revolutionized eye care and earned them recognition as visionary thinkers.

As the centuries unfolded, the knowledge and practices of medicine in the Arab Peninsula continued to evolve and adapt to discoveries and influences. The Arab world became a bridge between East and West, a conduit for the exchange of medical knowledge that enriched the global understanding of health and healing.

Today, the legacy of Arab medicine lives on, not only in the ancient texts and historical accounts but also in the modern practices and advancements in healthcare throughout the Arab world. The Arab Peninsula's rich history of medicine serves as a testament to the enduring human pursuit of healing and the remarkable ability of cultures to shape and contribute to the vast tapestry of medical knowledge that spans the globe.

Persian Medicine and Physicians:

Persian medicine, also known as Iranian traditional medicine or Unani medicine, is a system of healing that has been practiced in Iran for thousands of years. It is based on ancient Persian and Greek medical traditions and incorporates elements of Ayurveda and traditional Chinese medicine.

Persian medicine views the human body as a microcosm of the universe, with everyone being a unique combination of the four elements: earth, air, fire, and water. Health is achieved by maintaining a balance between these elements and the four humors: blood, phlegm, yellow bile, and black bile.

Practitioners of Persian medicine diagnose illnesses by considering various factors, including the patient's symptoms, pulse, urine analysis, and examination of the tongue. Treatment methods may include herbal remedies, dietary changes, detoxification, cupping, massage, and lifestyle modifications.

The principles of Persian medicine emphasize the prevention of disease by promoting a healthy lifestyle, proper nutrition, and maintaining a harmonious balance within the body. It also recognizes the importance of the mind-body connection and the role of emotions in overall health.

Today, Persian medicine continues to be practiced alongside modern medicine in Iran and other parts of the world. It has gained recognition for its holistic approach and its focus on individualized treatment. Research is ongoing to explore the scientific basis of Persian medicine and its potential integration with modern healthcare practices.

Persian and Iranian physicians have made significant contributions to the field of medicine throughout history. Numerous renowned Persian scholars and physicians have left a lasting impact on medical knowledge and practice.

One of the most famous Persian physicians is Avicenna (Ibn Sina), who lived in the 10th and 11th centuries. His medical encyclopedia, "The Canon of Medicine," became a renowned medical textbook in Europe and the Islamic world for several centuries. Avicenna's work covered various aspects of medicine, including anatomy, physiology, pathology, and pharmacology.

Another influential Persian physician is Rhazes (Al-Razi), who lived in the 9th and 10th centuries. He made significant contributions to the fields of pediatrics, ophthalmology, and neurology. Rhazes also introduced the concept of clinical observation and emphasized the importance of medical ethics in his writings.

In more recent times and before the 1979 Iranian Islamic takeover, Iranian physicians contributed to medical research and practice alongside the international medical communities.

Furthermore, Iran has a strong medical education system and is home to many reputable medical schools and research institutions. Iranian physicians are trained in both modern medicine and traditional medicine, allowing for a comprehensive approach to healthcare.

Overall, Persian and Iranian physicians have played a crucial role in advancing medical knowledge and practice, both in ancient times and in the present day. Their contributions have had a profound impact on the development of medicine globally.

Ancient Medicine:

In the ever-evolving landscape of modern medicine, the applicability of ancient and herbal medicine to complex disease processes has become a subject of great interest and debate. While medical advancements have undoubtedly revolutionized the way we approach and treat complex diseases, there is a growing recognition of the potential benefits that ancient practices and herbal remedies can offer in complementing modern treatments.

Ancient medicine, rooted in the wisdom of civilizations such as the Egyptians, Greeks, and Chinese, was often based on holistic approaches that considered the interconnectedness of the body, mind, and spirit. These ancient healers recognized the importance of balance, harmony, and the body's innate ability to heal itself.

In today's medicine, where complex diseases often require multifaceted approaches, the holistic perspective offered by ancient medicine can be invaluable. While modern medicine focuses on treating specific symptoms and diseases, ancient practices emphasize the importance of addressing the underlying causes and supporting the body's natural healing mechanisms.

Herbal medicine, derived from plants and natural substances, has also gained prominence in the field of modern medicine. Many pharmaceutical drugs have their roots in herbal remedies, with active ingredients isolated and synthesized for targeted treatments. However, the use of whole plant extracts and traditional herbal preparations is also gaining recognition for their potential therapeutic benefits.

Scientific research has shown that certain herbal remedies possess medicinal properties that can aid in the management of complex diseases. For example, the use of turmeric, a spice with anti-inflammatory properties, has shown promise in alleviating symptoms of conditions like arthritis and inflammatory bowel disease. Similarly, herbal preparations containing St. John's Wort have been studied for their potential antidepressant effects.

Moreover, ancient and herbal medicine offers an alternative for individuals who may not tolerate or respond well to conventional pharmaceuticals. In cases where patients experience adverse effects or lack of efficacy with modern treatments, complementary and alternative approaches based on ancient practices can provide viable options.

However, it is crucial to approach the integration of ancient and herbal medicine into modern healthcare with caution. While these practices can offer potential benefits, they must be subjected to rigorous scientific scrutiny. Robust research studies and clinical trials are necessary to establish their safety, efficacy, and optimal use in complex disease processes.

Furthermore, it is essential to recognize that ancient and herbal medicine should not replace modern medical interventions or discourage individuals from seeking appropriate care. Rather, they should be viewed as complementary tools that can enhance overall well-being and support the body's healing processes.

In this era of modern medicine, where technological advancements and pharmaceutical breakthroughs dominate the landscape, there is a growing realization that ancient and herbal medicine can offer valuable insights and therapeutic options for complex disease processes. By combining the best of both worlds - the knowledge and advancements of modern medicine with the time-tested wisdom of ancient practices and herbal remedies - we can pave the way for a more comprehensive and holistic approach to healthcare.

Herbal Medicine:

Herbal and home remedies have been used for centuries in the treatment of various ailments, including cancer and cardiovascular diseases. While modern medicine has made significant advancements in these fields, the role of herbal and home remedies in supporting conventional treatments and managing symptoms cannot be ignored.

In the case of cancer, herbal remedies have been studied for their potential anti-cancer properties and ability to alleviate side effects of treatments such as chemotherapy and radiation therapy. For instance, compounds derived from plants like turmeric, green tea, and garlic have shown promising anti-cancer effects in laboratory studies. These natural substances possess antioxidant and anti-inflammatory properties that may help inhibit the growth of cancer cells and reduce the risk of metastasis.

Additionally, herbal remedies such as ginger and peppermint have been used to alleviate nausea and vomiting, common side effects of chemotherapy. These natural remedies can provide relief and improve the quality of life for cancer patients undergoing aggressive treatments.

However, it is important to note that herbal remedies should never be used as a substitute for conventional cancer treatments. They should be seen as complementary approaches that can support the overall well-being of patients and potentially enhance the effectiveness of conventional therapies.

In the case of cardiovascular diseases, herbal and home remedies have also shown promise in managing symptoms and reducing the risk of complications. For example, the use of garlic has been associated with lowering blood pressure and cholesterol levels. Hawthorn extract, derived from the hawthorn plant, has been used traditionally to support heart health and improve circulation.

Moreover, lifestyle changes and home remedies can play a significant role in preventing and managing cardiovascular diseases. Regular exercise, a healthy diet rich in fruits and vegetables and stress reduction techniques like meditation and yoga can all contribute to cardiovascular health.

However, it is crucial to consult with healthcare professionals before incorporating herbal and home remedies into the treatment of cancer or cardiovascular diseases. They can guide the appropriate use, and potential interactions with medications, and ensure that these remedies do not interfere with the efficacy of prescribed treatments.

Furthermore, it is important to recognize that scientific evidence supporting the use of herbal and home remedies in cancer and cardiovascular diseases is still evolving. While some studies have shown positive effects, more research is needed to establish their safety, efficacy, and optimal dosages.

In summary, herbal and home remedies can play a supportive role in the treatment of cancer and cardiovascular diseases. They may help alleviate symptoms, reduce the side effects of treatments, and improve overall well-being. However, their use should always be discussed with healthcare professionals to ensure proper integration with conventional and modern therapies.

Islamic vs Modern Medicine: Islamic Medicine vs. Modern Medicine and Technology: Bridging the Gap for Better Healthcare Islamic medicine and modern medicine represent two distinct approaches to healthcare, each with its principles and methodologies. While modern medicine relies heavily on technological advancements and evidence-based practices, Islamic medicine draws from the teachings of the Quran and the traditions of the Prophet Muhammad (peace be upon him). This narrative explores the differences and similarities between Islamic medicine and modern medicine, highlighting the potential for bridging the gap to achieve better healthcare outcomes.

Islamic Medicine:

Islamic medicine is rooted in the belief that health and well-being are gifts from God and that the body possesses a natural ability to heal itself. It emphasizes holistic care, focusing not only on physical health but also spiritual, mental, and emotional well-being. Islamic medicine incorporates various practices such as herbal remedies, cupping therapy, and prophetic medicine, which refers to treatments and practices mentioned in the teachings of Prophet Muhammad (peace be upon him).

Modern Medicine and Technology:

Modern medicine, on the other hand, relies heavily on scientific research, evidence-based practices, and technological advancements. It places a strong emphasis on diagnosing and treating diseases using pharmaceuticals, surgeries, and medical devices. Technology has revolutionized modern medicine, enabling accurate diagnoses, advanced surgical procedures, and improved patient monitoring. From medical imaging to telemedicine, technology plays a crucial role in delivering quality healthcare services.

Bridging the Gap:

While Islamic medicine and modern medicine may seem divergent, there are opportunities for bridging the gap to achieve better healthcare outcomes. Islamic principles of holistic care align with the growing recognition of the importance of addressing both physical and mental health in modern medicine. Integrating spiritual and emotional well-being into healthcare practices can contribute to enhanced patient-centered care.

Furthermore, modern medicine can benefit from incorporating certain aspects of Islamic medicine. For example, herbal remedies and traditional practices can be explored for potential therapeutic benefits, and cupping therapy has been recognized for its potential in pain management. Collaborative research between Islamic scholars and medical professionals can help identify effective traditional treatments and validate their efficacy using modern scientific methods.

Additionally, the ethical principles emphasized in Islamic medicine, such as compassion, honesty, and respect for human dignity, can contribute to enhancing the doctor-patient relationship and patient satisfaction in modern healthcare settings. By incorporating these principles, modern medicine can prioritize patient-centered care and improve overall healthcare experiences.

Islamic medicine and modern medicine represent two distinct approaches to healthcare, each with its strengths and limitations. While modern medicine relies on technological advancements and evidence-based practices, Islamic medicine emphasizes holistic care and draws from religious teachings. By bridging the gap between these two approaches, healthcare providers can achieve better outcomes by integrating holistic care, exploring traditional treatments, and incorporating ethical principles into modern medical practices. Ultimately, a collaborative and inclusive approach to healthcare can lead to improved patient well-being and satisfaction.

Religious Medicine:

Once upon a time, in a small village nestled deep within the mountains, there lived a wise and respected healer named Amina. Amina was not only known for her extensive knowledge of herbal remedies but also her deep connection to the spiritual realm. She believed that healing was not only a physical process but also a spiritual one, and she incorporated both aspects into her practice.

The villagers sought Amina's help whenever they fell ill or faced any kind of ailment. They believed in her abilities to not only cure their physical ailments but also to ward off any evil spirits that might be causing their suffering. Amina's methods were a blend of religious and superstitious practices, rooted in the ancient traditions passed down through generations. She would recite prayers and perform rituals to invoke the blessings of the gods and goddesses, seeking their divine intervention in the healing process.

One day, a young woman named Leila came to Amina seeking a cure for a mysterious illness that had plagued her for months. Leila had visited numerous doctors and healers, but none had been able to offer her any relief. Desperate and losing hope, she turned to Amina for help.

Amina listened attentively as Leila described her symptoms, and then she began her examination. She carefully observed Leila's body, searching for any signs that might provide clues to the root cause of her illness. After a thorough examination, Amina concluded that Leila's ailment was not purely physical but had a spiritual component as well.

Amina asked Leila about her recent experiences and any possible encounters with negative energies. Leila revealed that she had recently moved into a new home, which had a reputation for being haunted. She had dismissed the rumors as mere superstitions, but now she wondered if there was any truth to them.

Amina nodded knowingly and explained that sometimes, physical illnesses could be manifestations of spiritual disturbances. She believed that negative energies could invade a person's body and cause harm. Amina decided to perform a ritual to cleanse Leila's spirit and restore her health.

Under the shimmering moonlight, Amina gathered the necessary herbs, candles, and sacred objects. She created a sacred space and began chanting ancient prayers, calling upon the spirits for guidance and protection. Amina then gently placed her hands on Leila's forehead and murmured incantations, invoking the healing powers of the gods.

As Amina performed the ritual, Leila felt a warm and comforting energy enveloping her. She closed her eyes, allowing herself to surrender to the healing process. Gradually, she felt a sense of peace and relief wash over her as if a weight had been lifted from her shoulders.

Days turned into weeks, and Leila's health steadily improved. Under Amina's care, the physical symptoms vanished, and Leila's spirit was rejuvenated. She could not thank Amina enough for her wisdom, her compassion, and her unwavering belief in the power of religious and superstitious medicine.

The word of Amina's healing powers spread throughout the region, and people from distant villages began seeking her help. Amina continued to combine her extensive knowledge of herbal remedies with her deep spiritual connection to provide relief to those in need.

In this small corner of the world, religious and superstitious medicine thrived, offering hope and solace to those who turned to it. Amina's legacy lived on, reminding people of the power of faith, spirituality, and the interconnectedness of the physical and spiritual realms.

Religious Medicine:

The Dark Side of Religious Medicine: Exploring the Dangers and Pitfalls

Religious medicine, with its deep-rooted beliefs and practices, has been a part of human society for centuries. From faith healing to spiritual rituals, this form of healing has provided solace and hope to countless individuals. However, it is essential to acknowledge that while religious medicine may offer comfort to some, there is a dark side to its practice that should not be overlooked. In this section, I will delve into the potential dangers and pitfalls of religious medicine.

1. Delayed or Inadequate Medical Treatment:

One of the significant risks associated with religious medicine is the potential for individuals to forgo or delay seeking proper medical treatment. In some cases, fervent believers may rely solely on religious remedies or practices, neglecting conventional medical advice. This can lead to worsened conditions, unnecessary suffering, and even fatalities that could have been prevented with timely medical intervention.

2. False Hope and Misinformation:

Religious medicine often promises miraculous results and healing through divine intervention. While faith can play a positive role in the healing process, it can also foster false hope and perpetuate misinformation. Individuals may be led to believe that they can be cured solely through prayer, rituals, or religious practices, without considering the scientific evidence or seeking appropriate medical help. This can lead to disappointment, a loss of trust in medical professionals, and the perpetuation of harmful beliefs.

3. Exploitation and Financial Burdens:

The practice of religious medicine has also been exploited by individuals seeking personal gain or financial profit. Charlatans and unscrupulous practitioners may take advantage of vulnerable individuals by offering expensive religious remedies or services that have no proven efficacy. This not only leads to financial burdens on already struggling individuals but also perpetuates a cycle of exploitation and deceit.

4. Reinforcement of Social Stigma:

In certain religious communities, the use of traditional or superstitious remedies may be strongly encouraged or enforced. This can create a social stigma around seeking conventional medical help, leading to ostracization or condemnation for those who choose to do so. This stigma can have severe consequences, particularly for individuals suffering from mental health issues or chronic illnesses, who may desperately require professional medical assistance.

5. Lack of Regulation and Accountability:

Unlike conventional medicine, religious medicine often operates outside the realm of regulatory bodies and quality control mechanisms. This lack of oversight can leave individuals vulnerable to ineffective or potentially harmful treatments. Without standardized practices, qualifications, or ethical guidelines, religious medicine can become a breeding ground for unqualified practitioners and questionable practices that put people's health at risk.

Religious medicine, with its deep spiritual beliefs and practices, can be a source of solace and hope for many individuals. However, it is crucial to recognize and address the dark side of this form of healing. The dangers and pitfalls associated with religious medicine, such as delayed medical treatment, misinformation, exploitation, social stigma, and a lack of regulation, cannot be ignored. By promoting a balanced approach that combines faith with evidence-based healthcare, we can ensure the well-being and safety of individuals seeking healing and medical assistance.

Islamic Republic of Iran and Covid-!9 Pandemic:

In a surprising turn of events, the Islamic Republic of Iran, under the leadership of Ayatollah Khamenei, has decided to halt the import of COVID-19 vaccines from the United States. This decision has sparked debate and curiosity among global observers, as it goes against the trend of many countries seeking to secure effective vaccines to combat the ongoing pandemic. In this part, I will delve into the possible reasons behind Iran's choice, analyze its potential implications, and discuss whether it is a prudent move or a missed opportunity.

National Sovereignty and Self-Sufficiency:

One of the key factors motivating Iran's decision could be its desire to assert national sovereignty and self-sufficiency. The Islamic Republic has often taken pride in its ability to resist external pressures and sanctions, and this decision might be seen as a reflection of that sentiment. By opting to rely on domestic resources and indigenous vaccine development, Iran aims to demonstrate its ability to overcome challenges independently.

Regional Politics and Geopolitical Considerations:

Iran has had a complex relationship with the United States, marked by decades of tension and strained diplomatic ties. This decision may be viewed within the context of ongoing regional politics and Iran's desire to reduce dependencies on foreign powers, particularly those with which it has had contentious relationships. By refusing to import vaccines from the US, Iran could be signaling its intent to establish alternative alliances and partnerships to ensure access to vaccines.

Supporting Domestic Vaccine Development:

Another potential reason behind Iran's decision is its commitment to supporting its domestic vaccine development efforts. Like many other countries, Iran has been investing in research and development to produce its own COVID-19 vaccines. By focusing on these efforts, Iran aims to not only address its own population's needs but also potentially contribute to global vaccination efforts in the future. However, over the past few years, Iran failed to manufacture any COVID-19 vaccine and continued importing less effective manufactured vaccines from Russia and China.

Possible Implications:

While Iran's decision to halt vaccine imports from the US may have been driven by various factors, it is crucial to assess the potential implications. Delaying access to vaccines, especially those proven effective through rigorous trials may pose risks to public health. The decision could potentially prolong the pandemic's impact on Iran's population, as well as hinder the country's ability to fully reopen its economy and resume normalcy.

Seeking International Cooperation:

Given the global nature of the pandemic, international cooperation and collaboration are vital in defeating COVID-19. Iran's decision to halt vaccine imports from the US may be an opportunity missed to partake in the global effort and benefit from the collective scientific knowledge and resources available. By actively engaging with international partners, Iran could not only secure vaccines but also contribute to the overall research and development of effective vaccines and treatments.

Iran's decision to halt the import of COVID-19 vaccines from the United States raises intriguing questions about national sovereignty, self-sufficiency, and regional politics. While it is an assertive move, it also carries potential risks for public health and the country's ability to combat the pandemic effectively. As the world strives to overcome this global crisis, fostering international cooperation and relying on proven scientific advancements are crucial. Iran's choice may yet be reconsidered as the situation evolves, and it remains to be seen how this decision will impact the nation's fight against COVID-19 in the future.

The Dark Chapter: Nazi Germany's Prohibition of Vaccination

The era of Nazi Germany, under the dictatorship of Adolf Hitler, is remembered as one of the darkest periods in human history. Alongside their heinous acts, the Nazis made a sinister decision to forbid vaccination within their regime. In this narrative, I will explore the reasons behind this prohibition, the historic outcomes, and the lasting impacts it had on public health.

The Prohibition of Vaccination:

In the early years of Nazi rule, the regime sought to exert control over all aspects of German society, including healthcare. They propagated an ideology that rejected established medical practices, including vaccination. Nazi leaders, including Hitler himself, believed in pseudoscientific theories that claimed vaccines were harmful, ineffective, and part of a larger conspiracy by Jewish doctors and pharmaceutical companies.

Consequences on Public Health:

The prohibition of vaccination had devastating consequences on public health in Nazi Germany. Preventable diseases, which vaccines could have effectively controlled, began to spread rapidly throughout the population. Measles, pertussis, diphtheria, and polio resurged, leading to increased illness, disability, and death. The most vulnerable members of society, such as children and the elderly, suffered the most.

Propaganda and Misinformation:

To enforce their anti-vaccination policy, the Nazis employed propaganda and disseminated misinformation. State-controlled media outlets and Nazi propaganda machinery spread messages claiming that vaccines were toxic and part of a larger conspiracy against the German people. Such false narratives further fueled public distrust in vaccines and the medical community, leading to widespread vaccine hesitancy.

Impact on Future Generations:

The long-term consequences of the Nazi regime's prohibition of vaccination are still felt today. The lack of vaccination during that period resulted in a generation of individuals who were not adequately immunized against various diseases. Even after the fall of the Nazi regime, Germany faced ongoing challenges in rebuilding its healthcare system and restoring public trust in vaccines.

Lessons Learned:

The prohibition of vaccination in Nazi Germany serves as a grim reminder of the dangers of pseudoscience, propaganda, and the suppression of established medical practices. It highlights the importance of evidence-based medicine, rigorous scientific research, and the need to trust reputable healthcare professionals.

Post-War Rebuilding:

After World War II and the defeat of Nazi Germany, the country embarked on a journey of rebuilding and reconciling with its troubled past. Part of this process involved reviving the healthcare system and reintroducing vaccination programs. Germany, like many other countries, recognized the immense value of vaccines in safeguarding public health and preventing the resurgence of preventable diseases.

The prohibition of vaccination in Nazi Germany stands as a tragic testament to the dangers of misinformation, propaganda, and the suppression of medical advancements. The consequences of the regime's decision to forbid vaccination were severe, leading to the spread of preventable diseases and untold suffering. We must learn from this dark chapter in history, ensuring that evidence-based medicine and the benefits of vaccines are never compromised or denied.

Prohibition of COVID-19 Vaccine in the Islamic Republic of Iran:

Ayatollah Khamenei's Controversial Decision: The Prohibition of the COVID-19 Vaccine In recent times, the world has faced the unprecedented challenge of the COVID-19 pandemic. While nations worldwide have been striving to combat the virus, a controversy arose when Ayatollah Ali Khamenei, the Supreme Leader of Iran, announced a prohibition on the COVID-19 vaccine. This narrative delves into the reasons behind this decision, the historic outcomes, and the potential ramifications it may have on public health.

The Prohibition of the COVID-19 Vaccine:

In January 2021, Ayatollah Khamenei made a surprising announcement, rejecting the importation and use of the COVID-19 vaccines produced by Western countries. Citing unfounded claims that the vaccines could be used as a tool for foreign infiltration or that they might not be trustworthy, the Supreme Leader instated a policy against the vaccination campaign within Iran.

Consequences on Public Health:

The prohibition of the COVID-19 vaccine by Ayatollah Khamenei has had significant consequences on public health within Iran. Despite the country being severely impacted by the pandemic, with thousands of lives lost and a strained healthcare system, the decision to forbid vaccination has hindered the nation's ability to protect its citizens from the virus. The lack of vaccination has allowed COVID-19 to continue to spread, leading to increased illness, hospitalizations, and fatalities.

Public Mistrust and Misinformation:

Ayatollah Khamenei's decision exacerbated public mistrust in the COVID-19 vaccine. The prohibition became a catalyst for the spread of misinformation and conspiracy theories surrounding the vaccine's safety and efficacy. This misinformation further fueled vaccine hesitancy, hindering efforts to mitigate the impact of the pandemic and protect public health.

International Response and Concerns:

The international community expressed deep concern over Ayatollah Khamenei's prohibition of the COVID-19 vaccine. Health experts and organizations emphasized the importance of widespread vaccination to control the virus globally. The decision by the Supreme Leader was seen as contradictory to these efforts, raising questions about Iran's commitment to international collaboration and public health.

Potential Long-Term Impacts:

The long-term impacts of the prohibition of the COVID-19 vaccine in Iran are yet to be fully realized. The continued spread of the virus within the country and the absence of vaccination leave the population vulnerable to ongoing health risks. Moreover, the decision's impact on public trust in the Iranian healthcare system and future vaccination campaigns may hinder the nation's ability to respond effectively to future health crises.

Lessons to Learn:

Ayatollah Khamenei's prohibition of the COVID-19 vaccine in Iran serves as a reminder of the dangers of politicizing public health measures. It underscores the importance of evidence-based decision-making, international collaboration, and trust in scientific advancements. The COVID-19 pandemic has demonstrated the critical role vaccines play in protecting public health, and any prohibition should be based on sound scientific evidence and expert consensus.

Ayatollah Khamenei's decision to prohibit the COVID-19 vaccine in Iran has had significant consequences on public health within the country. The lack of vaccination has hindered efforts to control the virus, leading to increased illness and fatalities. Lessons must be learned from this prohibition, emphasizing the importance of evidence-based decision-making and trust in scientific advancements to safeguard public health in the face of future challenges.

Covid-19 Related Deaths in Islamic Republic of Iran Statistics and Aftermath:

The outbreak of the COVID-19 pandemic has had a profound impact on countries around the world. The Islamic Republic of Iran has been no exception, experiencing a significant number of COVID-19-related deaths. This section sheds light on the statistics surrounding these fatalities and explores the aftermath of the pandemic on Iran's healthcare system and society.

The Statistics:

As of 2022, the Islamic Republic of Iran has reported a considerable number of COVID-19-related deaths. According to official figures, the death toll has surpassed 178000, and data from personal communication reveals more than 700000 COVID-19-related deaths, making Iran one of the countries most affected by the virus. However, it is important to note that these numbers may not fully reflect the true extent of COVID-19-related deaths due to underreporting or lack of testing in certain areas.

Impact on the Healthcare System:

The high number of COVID-19-related deaths has placed immense strain on Iran's healthcare system. Hospitals have been overwhelmed with patients, leading to shortages of critical medical supplies, beds, and healthcare personnel. The healthcare system struggled to cope with the influx of cases, resulting in limited access to quality care for many individuals. The aftermath of the pandemic has left the healthcare system grappling with the need for improved infrastructure and resources to prevent future crises.

Socioeconomic Consequences:

The COVID-19-related deaths in Iran have had far-reaching socioeconomic consequences.

The nationwide lockdowns and restrictions imposed to curb the spread of the virus have disrupted various industries, leading to job losses and economic instability. Many businesses, particularly small and medium-sized enterprises, have faced closures, exacerbated unemployment rates, and reduced household incomes. The aftermath of the pandemic has left a lasting impact on the country's economy and the livelihoods of its citizens.

Grief and Psychological Impact:

The loss of loved ones due to COVID-19 has caused immense grief and psychological distress within Iranian society. Families have been torn apart, and communities have mourned the loss of their members. The psychological impact of the pandemic, coupled with the challenges of accessing mental health services, has further strained individuals and communities. The aftermath of the pandemic calls for increased support and resources to address the psychological toll experienced by the Iranian population.

Government Response and Lessons Learned:

The Iranian government's response to the COVID-19-related deaths has been met with both praise and criticism. Efforts were made to implement preventive measures and provide healthcare services to those affected. However, there were instances of delayed decision-making and inconsistencies in messaging, which may have contributed to the spread of the virus. The aftermath of the pandemic necessitates a thorough evaluation of the government's response to better prepare for future health crises.

International Collaboration and Support:

The impact of COVID-19-related deaths in Iran has highlighted the importance of international collaboration and support. The country has sought assistance from international organizations and received aid from various countries to combat the virus. The aftermath of the pandemic emphasizes the need for continued global cooperation and sharing of resources to mitigate the adverse effects of future health emergencies.

COVID-19-related deaths in the Islamic Republic of Iran have had a profound impact on the country's healthcare system, economy, and society. The high number of fatalities has strained the healthcare system, leading to shortages and limited access to care. The socioeconomic consequences, coupled with the psychological toll on individuals and communities, further compound the challenges faced by Iran. The aftermath of the pandemic calls for enhanced support, government evaluation, and international collaboration to build resilience and better respond to future health crises.

Healthcare System
Twelve to eighteen months actionable project.

Health Policy:

Social determinants, location, housing, education, employment, income, crime, and social cohesion are factors that significantly impact community health which is directly intertwined with the country's GDP. Although not verifiable, IR's reported share of healthcare was 6% of GPD in 2017.

Healthcare and the well-being of a country directly influence social determinants and vice seas, one could adversely and negatively influence the other.

Short-term proposal after regime change:

The proposal is classified as immediate, the first 100 days to 18 months, and long-term; the five years of strategic planning.

Immediate actionable proposal, Primary Care Axis.

Primary Care is the backbone and one of the major pillars of healthcare systems. Primary care is divided into two tracks, centralized and decentralized.

It appears that for the first few months, a combined approach would be more fruitful in current poorly tangent healthcare system.

1- While effortlessly working on utilizing the existing primary health system, it is prudent to partner with international organizations such as.

A- International Healthcare Volunteers (IHCV)

B- Global Health Volunteers (GHV)

C- Volunteers in Asia

D- Doctors without Borders

E- Atlantis Fellowship

2- Temporary deregulation of Primary Care and Preventive Care.

Currently, there are 90000 certified physicians in Iran providing care to 85000000 Iranians.

Chronically the healthcare, primary care, preventive care, and overall health systems have been underperformed, mismanaged, and total failure.

There are some discrepancies in several medical students and residents in Iran, however, extrapolating from different sources, it appears there are 4000 medical graduates each year of them some will leave the country, and around 10-20 absorbed in residency programs.

A- Create a Knowledge-Based governance model, which provides and supports a time-bound and focused teams with a measurable outcome.

B- Budget.

Reprogram the formally allocated, total allocated budget (TAB), the TAB will satisfy the additional needs and performance. This will guarantee project success.

C- The short-term and initial phase will be decentralized Primary and preventive care. The specialized and hospital care would be on an aggressive and observed referral system which has been inefficient and failed in the past 44 years.

D- Task force structure:

Refer to as Clinical Activities:

Clinical Activities consist of:

1- All Tamin e Ejtemaaee across the country.

2- All Universities Health systems, hospitals, and

clinics. 3- All free and charity clinics

4- All private hospitals, multi-specialty clinics, and single private medical offices.

5- All military, Sepal e Pasdran, and foundations hospitals and clinics.

6- Red Cross (Red Crescent) facilities

7- Physicians, Nurses, Pharmacists, Allied health providers, First Aids and Emergency staff

(EMS).

8- Medical Students and Residents.

Task Force personnel:

All current personnel of the mentioned facilities and organizations

This Program is regional, state, and local run with emphasis on primary and preventive care. A special task force will be formed for rural and remote areas.

All care recipients will be identified by National Identification cards and numbers, for tracking, referral, and follow-up services.

Payment:

There will be a temporary TAB administered by task force leadership and will utilize the current Tamine e Ejtemaaee pay system already in place with some adjustments. The payment should be guaranteed and the fee for the service schedule should be established at a higher level based on the level of service. This incentivized payment to all providers should be planned for the duration of the initial phase.

To make this phase more attractive to all providers, there should be more incentives which later on, could be rolled over to a permanent program.

Incentive Programs.

1- Higher Pay schedules by distance, the distance would be calculated from the capitols, and counties ......, or could be population-based or a combination of distance and

population. 2- Loan forgiveness

3- Forfeiting military and obligatory licensing requirements for 2-5 years.

4- Credit to enter residency programs.

5- scholarship Program

6- Facilitate an exchange program.

7- facilitate and help to enter medical education/medical school for allied health providers and qualified and eligible staff.

8- Starter up professional loans.

Leadership:

The success of the clinical activities depends on “buy-in” from Iran's current healthcare
providers and leaders.

The task force team leaders should have special clearance and authority from a higher level of the transitional governing body.

The team members should commit to attending all scheduled training, refreshing courses, and all clinical activities and prescribed patient care.

All team members are leaders, providers, and influencers. Each team member represents the respective professional organization and transitional Iran transitional government and is accountable for their high-quality performance and responsibilities.

All team members are responsible for achieving the objectives of the program and transparency on their performance, reporting, and informing the public of their mission.

The leadership is responsible for implementing, managing, and operational and administrative issues from the time of inception to the completion of the project.

Experience, the lesson learned and the program components, tools, and procedures will provide groundwork transitioning to long-term health systems programs and policies.

About the Author

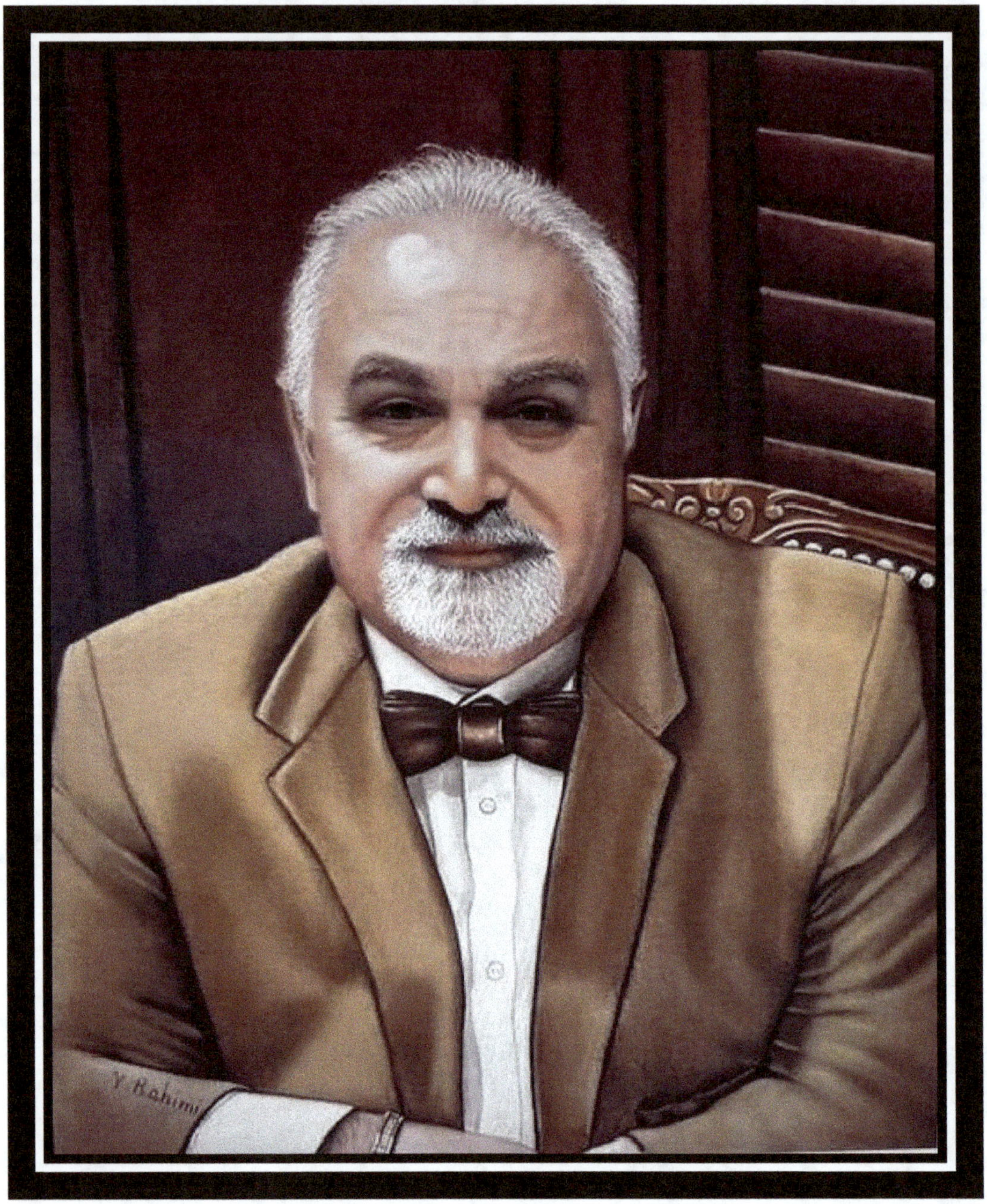

Ali R. Rahimi, M.D., FACP, AGSF

Dr. Rahimi received his medical degree and completed his internship at Ferdowsi University School of Medicine and Health Science Center in Iran. Upon graduation from medical school, he completed his residency training in Internal Medicine and a cardiology fellowship at St. Thomas' Hospital and Medical School in London, England.

Before relocating to the United States, Dr. Rahimi served as Chief of Cardiology at Labafi Nedjat Cardiovascular Medical Center in Iran. Subsequently, he joined Washington State

University in Pullman, Washington as a Research Assistant Professor in the Department of Physiology and Cardiovascular Sciences.

During his tenure with Washington State University, he worked on left ventricular function and mechanical properties. The result of his work was published in the American Journal of Pharmacology and Physiology. Dr. Rahimi continued his medical education domestically by completing residency training in Internal Medicine at St. Raphael Hospital, Yale University, and a fellowship in Geriatric Medicine at Duke University. Dr. Rahimi is Board Certified in Internal Medicine and Geriatric Medicine and served as Associate Program Director of Medical Education. Dr. Rahimi's passion for medicine motivated him to serve as Chief of Geriatric Medicine, Curriculum Chief for Geriatric and Behavior Medicine, and Director of Research and Scholarly activity at Mercer University Savannah Campus.

Dr. Rahimi's active career includes an elected Fellow in the American College of Physicians and American Geriatric Society, a Certified Medical Director for long-term care, and the primary investigator in more than 30 clinical trials over the past 20 years.

While it isn't the end of Dr. Rahimi's biography, he has authored or co-authored many scientific publications in Iran, England, and the United States, in addition to presentations to faculty at the American Geriatric Society, American Heart Association, Association of American Medical Colleges (AAMC) and Southern Medical Association (SMA), and American College of Physicians (ACP).

Dr. Rahimi is also a Certified Human Rights Consultant.

References and Citations

1. "Healthcare in Iran: An Overview" - World Health Organization (WHO)
2. "Healthcare System in Iran: Challenges and Opportunities" - Iranian Journal of Public Health
3. "Healthcare Expenditure and Financing in Iran" - International Journal of Health Policy and Management
4. "Healthcare Quality Assurance in Iran" - Journal of Medical Ethics and History of Medicine
5. "Healthcare Services in Iran: Achievements and Challenges" - Iranian Journal of Public Health
6. "Primary Healthcare in Iran: Challenges and Solutions" - Iranian Journal of Public Health
7. "Healthcare Workforce in Iran: Current Status and Future Challenges" - Iranian Journal of Public Health
8. "Healthcare Information Technology in Iran: Current Status and Future Directions" Health Information Management Journal
9. "Healthcare Financing in Iran: Achievements and Challenges" - Iranian Journal of Public Health
10. "Healthcare Equity in Iran: Progress and Challenges" - Iranian Journal of Public Health
11. "Healthcare in Iran: An Overview" by Arash Rashidian et al. (International Journal of Health Policy and Management, 2013)
12. "The Iranian healthcare system: An overview" by Mohammadreza Amiresmaili and Zahra Rezaei (Journal of Medical Systems, 2017)
13. "Healthcare system in Iran: An overview" by Elaheh Hooshmand and Mohammadreza Amiresmaili (Journal of Public Health Research, 2013)
14. "The Evolution of the Health Sector in Iran: An Overview" by Ali Akbari Sari et al.

(Annals of Global Health, 2014)
15. "Health Care in Iran" by Reza Malekzadeh and Reza Majdzadeh (Annals of Internal Medicine, 2019)
16. "The Iranian Health System in Transition" by Ali Akbari Sari et al. (International Journal of Health Policy and Management, 2014)
17. "The Technologists: How a Few Revolutionary Individuals Changed the World" by Matthew Pearl. This book explores the role of technologists throughout history in shaping the world and fighting against corrupt regimes.
18. "The Future of Technology: A Guide to Technocratic Governance" by Jason Pontin. This book discusses the potential of technology and technocratic governance in combating corruption and subversion.
19. "The Code Book: The Science of Secrecy from Ancient Egypt to Quantum Cryptography" by Simon Singh. This book delves into the history of cryptography and how it has been used to fight against corrupt regimes and subversion.
20. "The Idealist: Aaron Swartz and the Rise of Free Culture on the Internet" by Justin Peters. This book tells the story of Aaron Swartz, a technologist and activist who fought for transparency, open access, and against corruption.
21. "Technocracy: The Politics of Expertise" by Matthew A. Crenson and Benjamin Ginsberg. This book explores the concept of technocracy and its potential in challenging corrupt regimes and subversion.
22. The Age of Surveillance Capitalism: The Fight for a Human Future at the New Frontier of Power" by Shoshana Zuboff. This book discusses the impact of technology and surveillance capitalism on society and the fight against corruption and subversion.
23. "The Innovators: How a Group of Hackers, Geniuses, and Geeks Created the Digital Revolution" by Walter Isaacson. This book explores the history of technological innovation and the individuals who have fought against corruption and subversion through their inventions.
24. "The Man Behind the Microchip: Robert Noyce and the Invention of Silicon Valley"

by Leslie Berlin. This book tells the story of Robert Noyce, a pioneer of the microchip, and how his work contributed to the fight against corruption and subversion.

25. "The Black Box Society: The Secret Algorithms That Control Money and Information" by Frank Pasquale. This book examines the impact of algorithms and technology on society and the fight against corruption and subversion.
26. "The New Digital Age: Transforming Nations, Businesses, and Our Lives" by Eric Schmidt and Jared Cohen. This book explores the potential of technology to transform societies and fight against corruption and subversion.
27. "The Clean Coder: A Code of Conduct for Professional Programmers" by Robert C. Martin. This book provides guidance for technocrats and programmers on ethical practices and the fight against corruption and subversion in the tech industry.
28. "The Open Organization: Igniting Passion and Performance" by Jim Whitehurst. This book discusses the importance of open and transparent organizations in fighting against corruption and subversion in the technology sector.

www.ingramcontent.com/pod-product-compliance
Lightning Source LLC
LaVergne TN
LVHW080039210926
848481LV00011B/3232